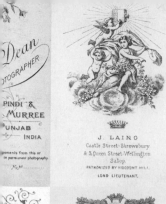
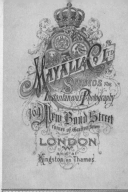
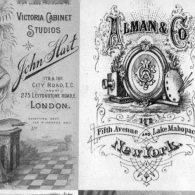
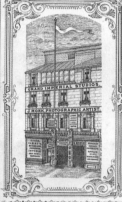

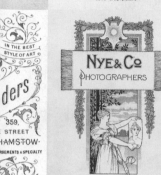
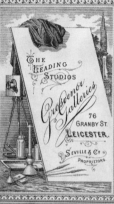
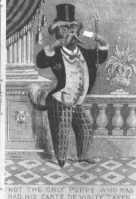
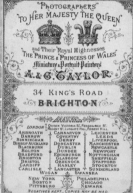
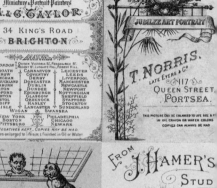

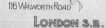
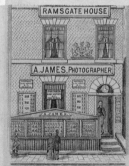
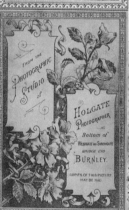
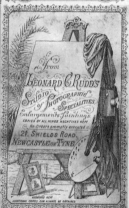
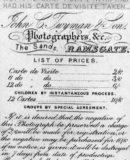
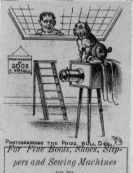

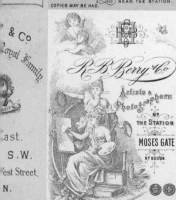
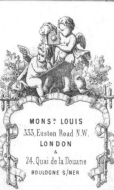
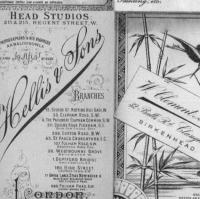
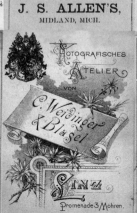
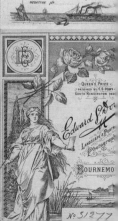

These Were Our Dogs

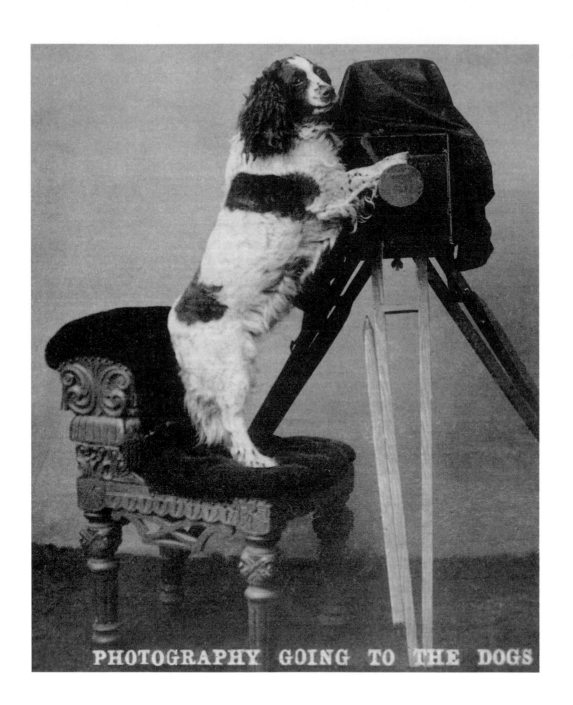

PHOTOGRAPHY GOING TO THE DOGS

These Were Our Dogs
Libby Hall

BLOOMSBURY

First published 2007

Copyright © 2007 by Libby Hall

The moral right of the author has been asserted

Bloomsbury Publishing Plc, 36 Soho Square, London W1D 3QY

A CIP catalogue record for this book is available from the British Library

ISBN 978 0 7475 8876 4
10 9 8 7 6 5 4 3 2 1

Designed by William Webb

Printed and bound by C&C Offset Printing CO., Ltd, China

www.bloomsbury.com

Contents

Dedicated to the men and women,
known and anonymous,
who took these photographs

and to the people and dogs
who posed for them.

Foreword

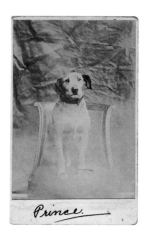

In 1966, when I first began collecting photographs of dogs, it was really just to save them, and other miscellaneous photographs, from being thrown into dustbins or destroyed on bonfires. (In those long-ago days dealers were more interested in the empty albums than they were in their contents.) Over the past forty years these random pictures have grown into a widely comprehensive and historically significant collection of dog photographs, but the collection has remained, inevitably, a highly personal and idiosyncratic selection.

There have been several excellent collections of early dog photographs published in the past twenty years. Those images have been gathered together from many sources, often by now-famous photographers, and those books give a fine feeling of the Dog as Art. The essence of this collection, however, lies in the fact that it represents a random, serendipitous assortment of images that have come into the field of view of one individual searcher.

These Were Our Dogs, together with my first three books, *Prince and Others*, *Prince II* and *Postcard Dogs*, is a testimony to the profound relationship that exists between Man and Dog as well as to the commonplace: to the ubiquitous image of Dog as Friend.

In the beginning I was simply rescuing photographs; then, a bit later, buying them from local flea markets and second-hand shops. Now they are finding their way to me from sources all over the world: from dealers who have become friends and know exactly what is likely to appeal to me, from international photographic fairs, and, of course, in the 21st century, from the all-encompassing internet auction sites. But the collection still has a *found* feel to it. I am still as likely to turn up what I consider a treasure in a local junk shop or flea market as I am from a high-powered international dealer.

I have never been concerned with 'antique' photographs as artefacts, as *objects*: only with the content of the image. Consequently I have been quite happy to buy pictures that have been in poor condition and to restore and repair them, something that would appal some collectors for whom the condition of the original photograph is all-important. But, while I have had no qualms about restoring a damaged image so that its content is easier to see, I have been scrupulous in not altering in any way the *essence* of an image.

With the magic available to modern restorers using software such as Photoshop, the reader is left with no choice but simply to trust the integrity of the restorer. I could, for instance, have added dogs to images that had no dogs! But in fact I have remained meticulously true to each original photograph.

As I said in the introduction to *Prince II*, 'Some reviewers of my earlier book of dog photographs... mentioned the lack of pedigreed dogs among my selection. This wasn't deliberate on my part. There were far fewer breeds of dog in the late nineteenth and early twentieth centuries. And the breeds that there were tended to be less extreme, less the result of human caprice, and consequently, in many cases, a great deal healthier and happier.' As time goes by I feel even more strongly that this is so, and I dream of a future where dogs are bred, not to satisfy arbitrary rules of cosmetic form, but, rather, to enhance their ability to function, and their subsequent good health and happiness.

The likely country of origin and, where known, information about the sitter, or notes from the back of the print, are given with each photograph. Other information is at the back of the book.

The photographs are in no particular chronological order. They range in date from approximately 1850 to 1940. I haven't attempted to date the images, except where I had specific information as to when they were taken.

For those readers who are interested in knowing more about the fascinating history of photography I have listed some excellent books in the short bibliography – as well as some fine books about dogs.

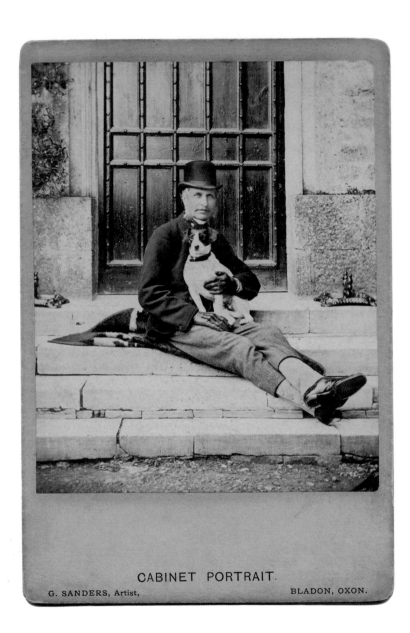

CABINET PORTRAIT.

G. SANDERS, Artist,   BLADON, OXON.

British

Note on reverse:
'Col Hon R. Spencer.
Woodstock. Probably
Colonel Hon Robert
Charles Henry Spencer
(1817 – 1881)'

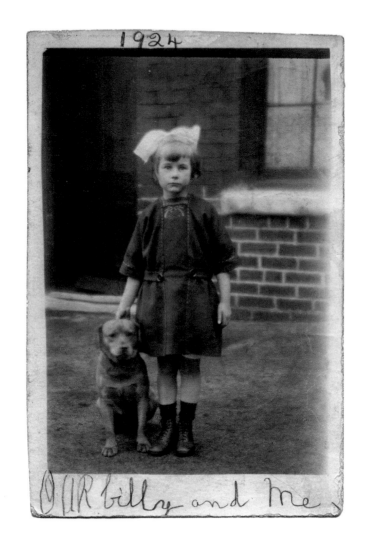

13

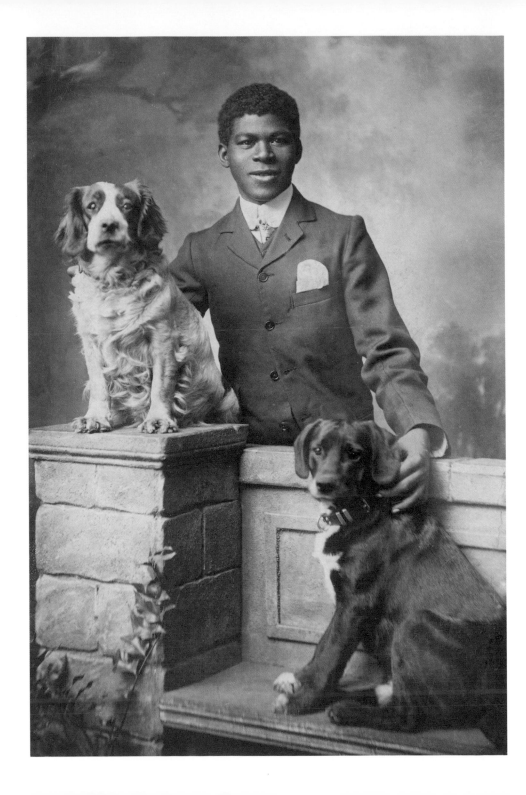

14

British

Postcard posted
from Clacton-on-
Sea to London,
September 1907:
'...this is the photo
of boots and
the dogs.'

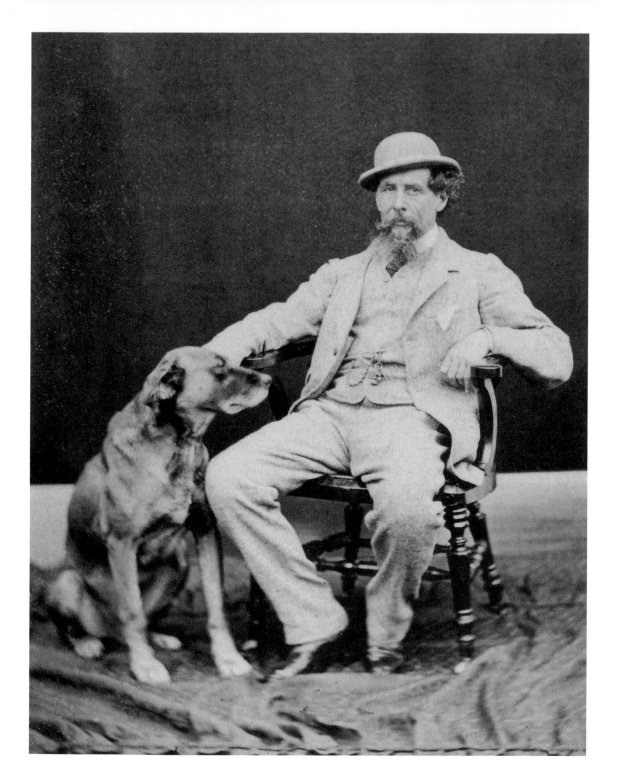

15

British

Charles Dickens
with his dog Turk.
Dickens and Turk
were known to
be devoted to
each other.

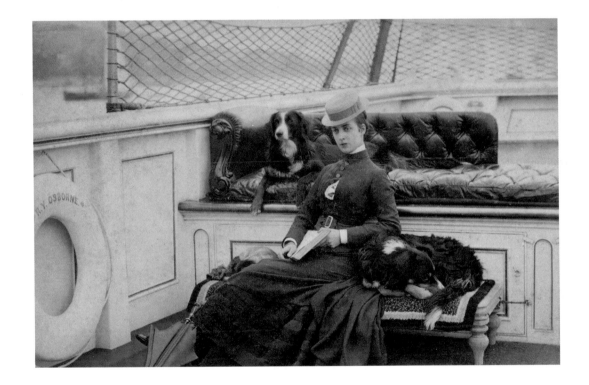

British

H.R.H. the Princess
of Wales and
favourite dogs on
board the royal
yacht *Osborne*.

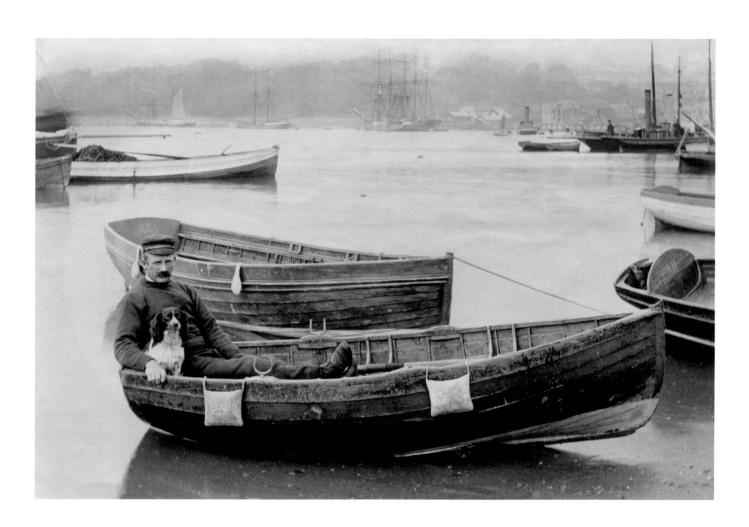

British

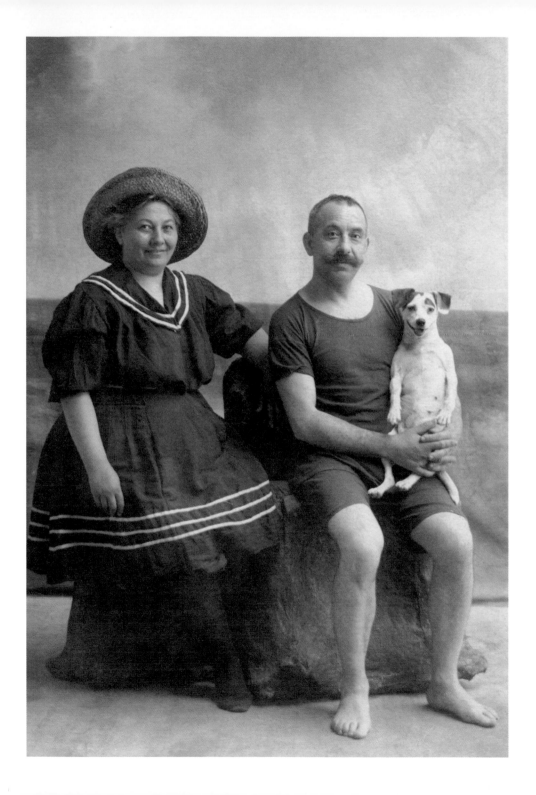

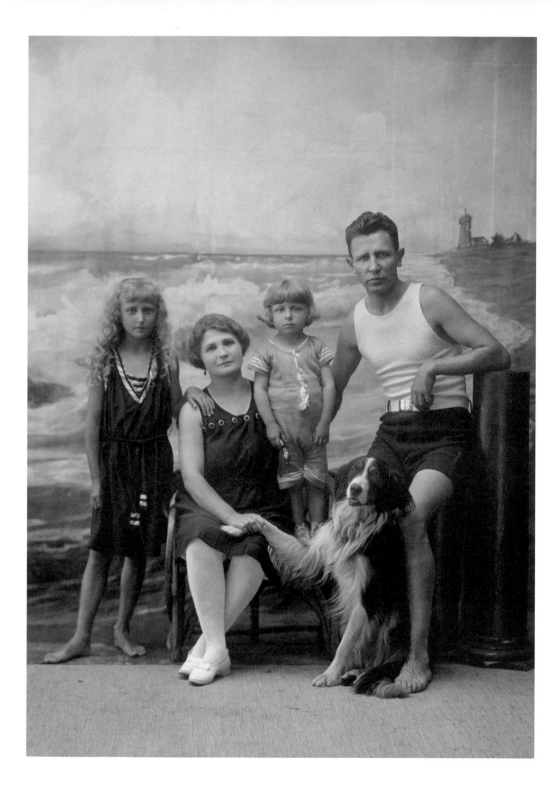

American

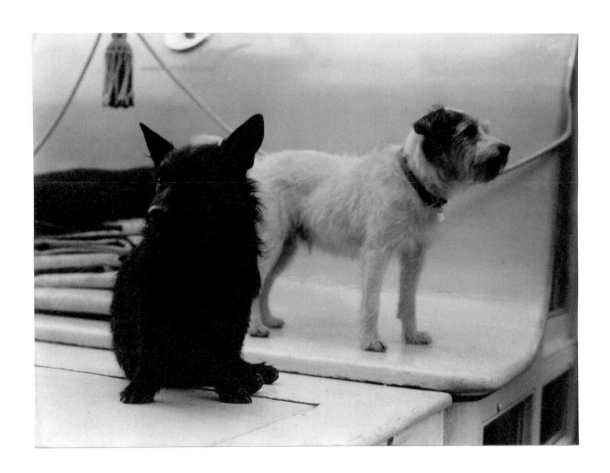

British

A previously unknown photograph, by
Queen Alexandra, of Princess Victoria's
constant companion, Mac, and Edward
VII's beloved Caesar. Taken on board
the Royal Yacht *Victoria and Albert*,
August 1908.

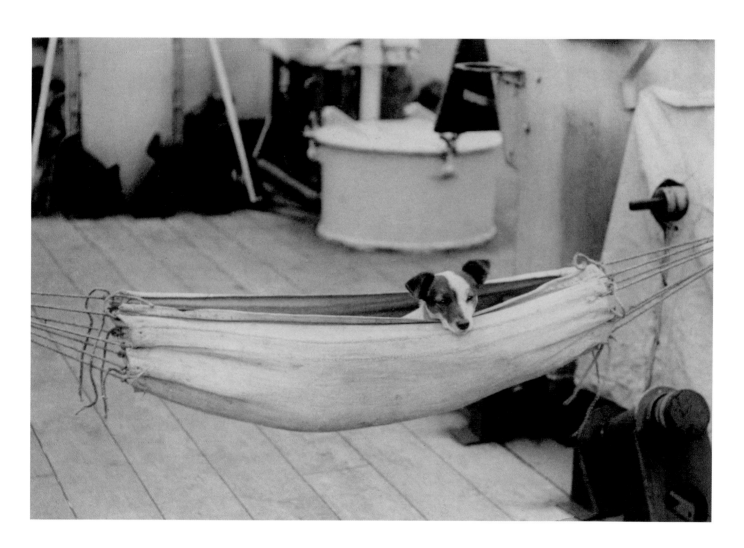

British

22

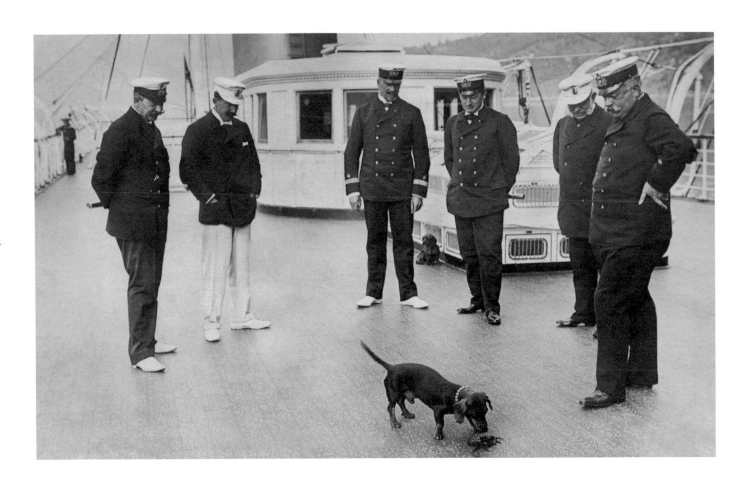

German

Der Kaiser mit seinem Lieblingshund Erdmann. One of a series of several photographs taken on the same occasion, which show a total of three dachshunds on deck. Only the Kaiser's darling dog, Erdmann, seems to have been given crab for lunch!

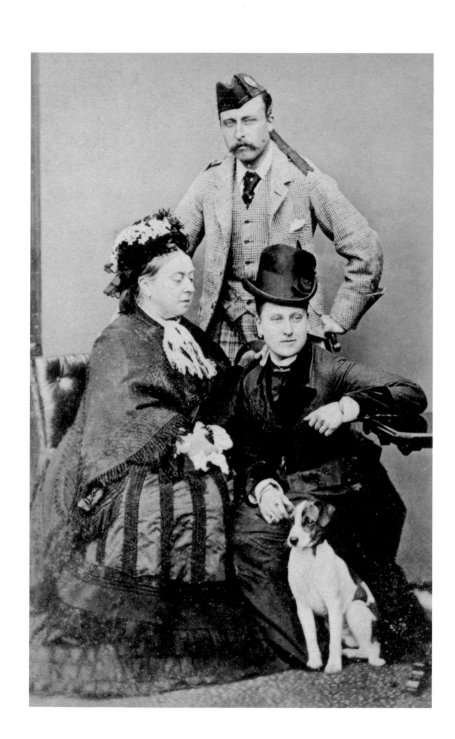

British

Queen Victoria,
Princess Beatrice,
the Duke of
Connaught and
Princess Beatrice's
dog, Wat.

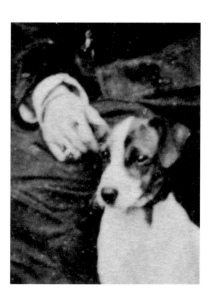

24

British

John Brown, Queen Victoria's personal servant, 1871.
Photographed by Hills and Saunders. The dogs are Corran,
Dächo, Rochie and Sharp. Sharp was one of the Queen's
favourite dogs and was photographed many times. He is also
the dog with her in the following photographs. He was born
in 1864 and died in 1879.

This print, taken from the original glass negative now in my
collection, is one of probably only two prints in existence, the
other being in the Royal Collection at Windsor.

Because the sitter's look and demeanour are so definitely not
that expected of a servant, this image would not have been
thought suitable to be sold to the public as a commercial
carte-de-visite, and it is probable that there were very few
prints ever made.

My thanks to all the photography curators in museums and
galleries who have looked for possible copies of this image.
Most particularly my thanks to the Royal Collection Trust
for allowing me to search for the photograph in Queen
Victoria's albums, and to Sophie Gordon, curator
of photographs, for her generous help.

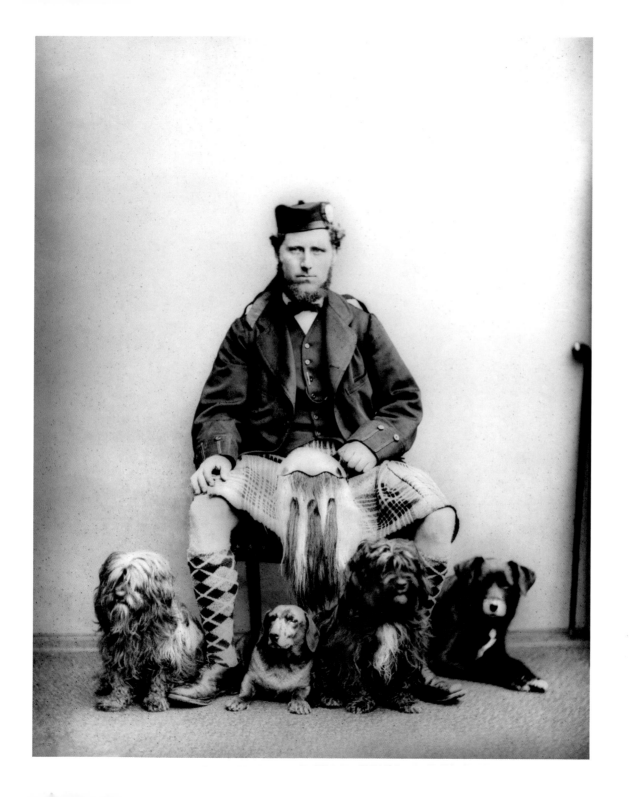

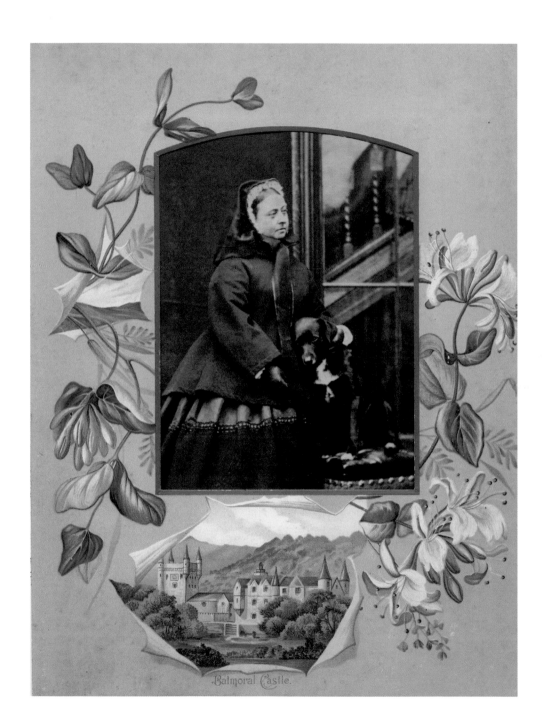

British

Queen Victoria
with her beloved
dog Sharp.
Balmoral, 1867.

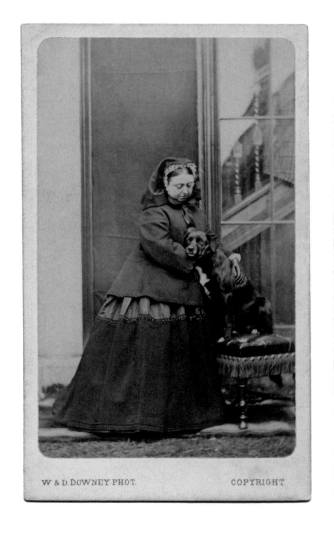

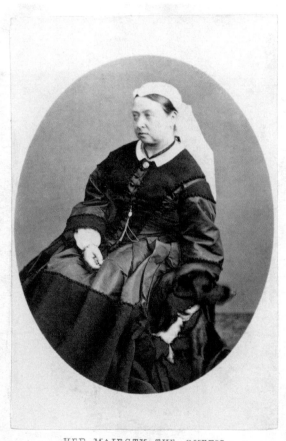

British

Queen Victoria
and Sharp.
Balmoral, 1867.

British

Queen Victoria
and Sharp.

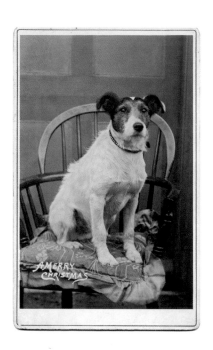

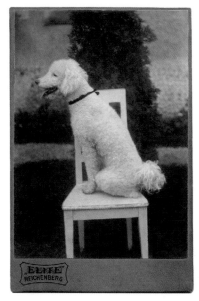

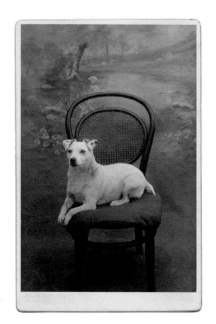

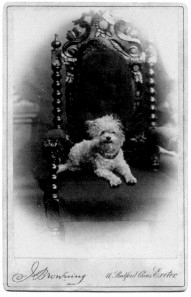

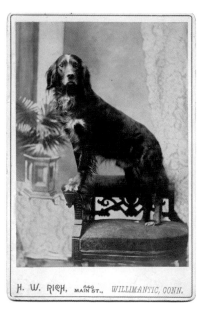

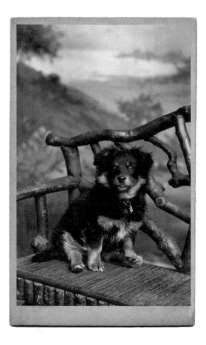

British

Bohemian

British

British

American

British

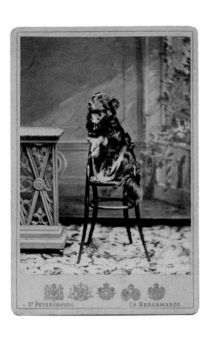

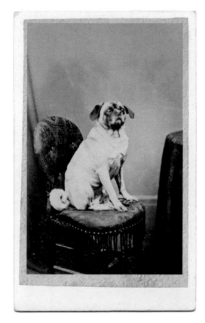

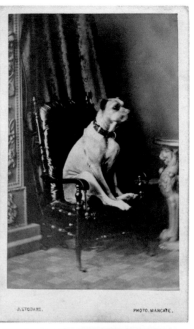

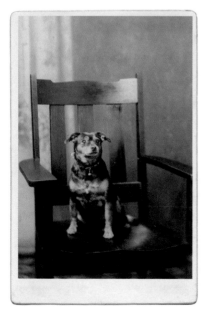

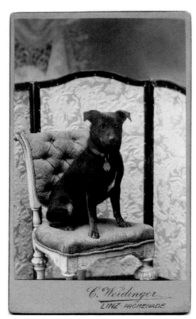

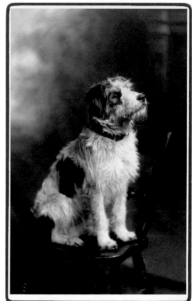

Russian

Probably American

British

Austrian

British

British

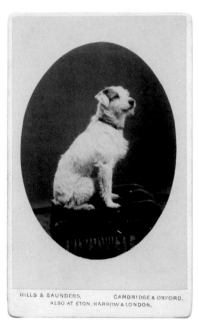

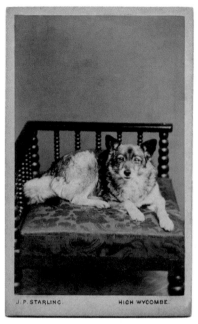

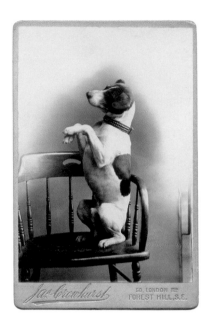

HILLS & SAUNDERS,   CAMBRIDGE & OXFORD.
ALSO AT ETON, HARROW & LONDON.

J. P. STARLING.   HIGH WYCOMBE.

Jas Crowhurst   50, LONDON R?
FOREST HILL, S.E.

30

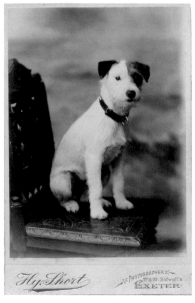

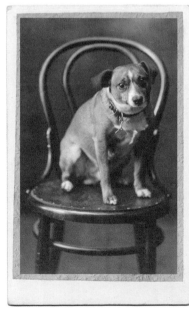

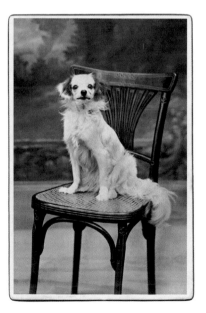

Hy Short   PHOTOGRAPHER
37 & St. Sidwell's
EXETER.

British   British   British

British   American   British

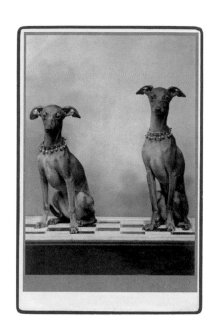

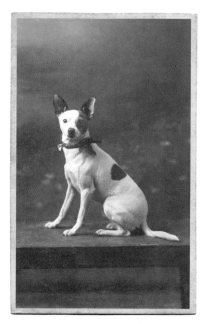

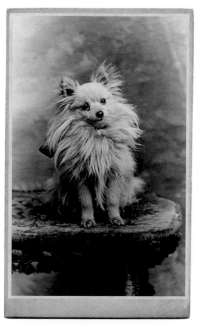

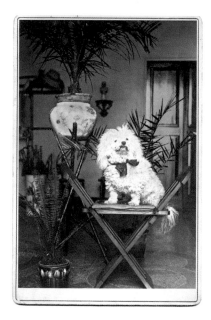

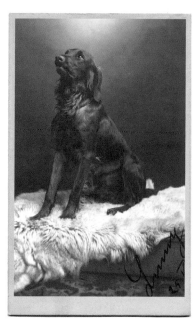

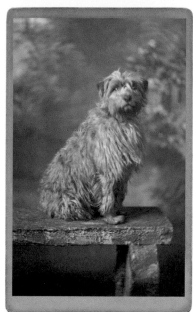

European

French

British

German

British

British

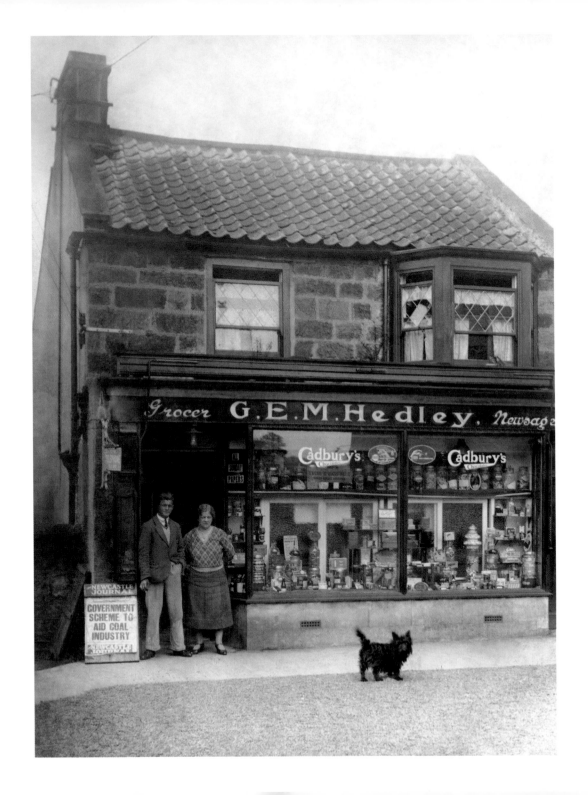

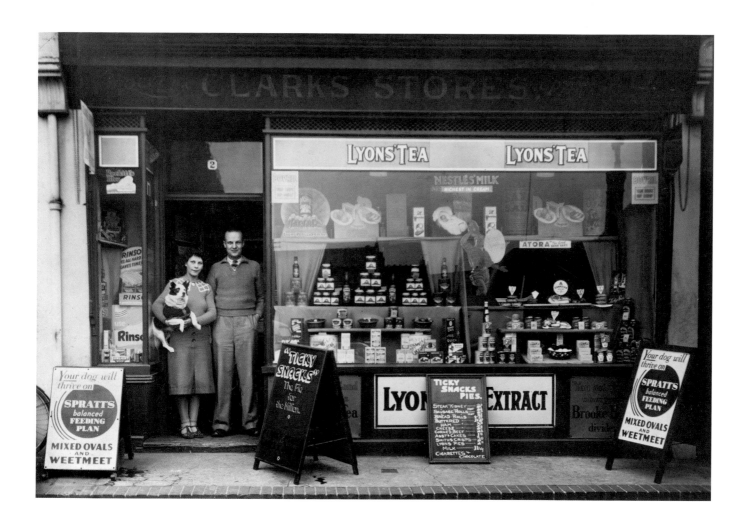

British

34

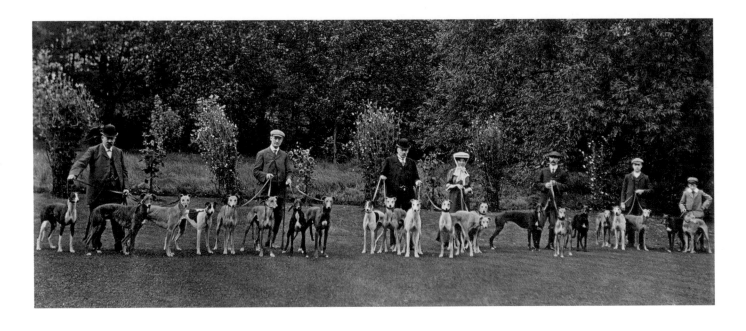

British

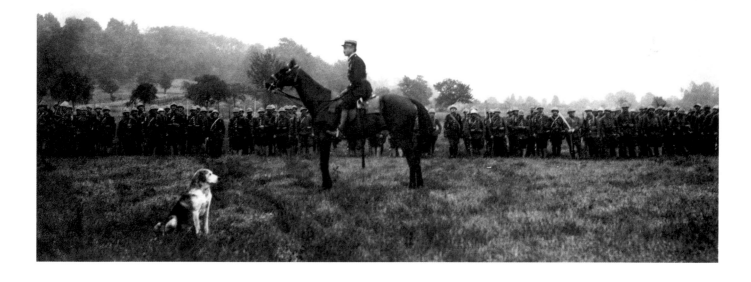

French

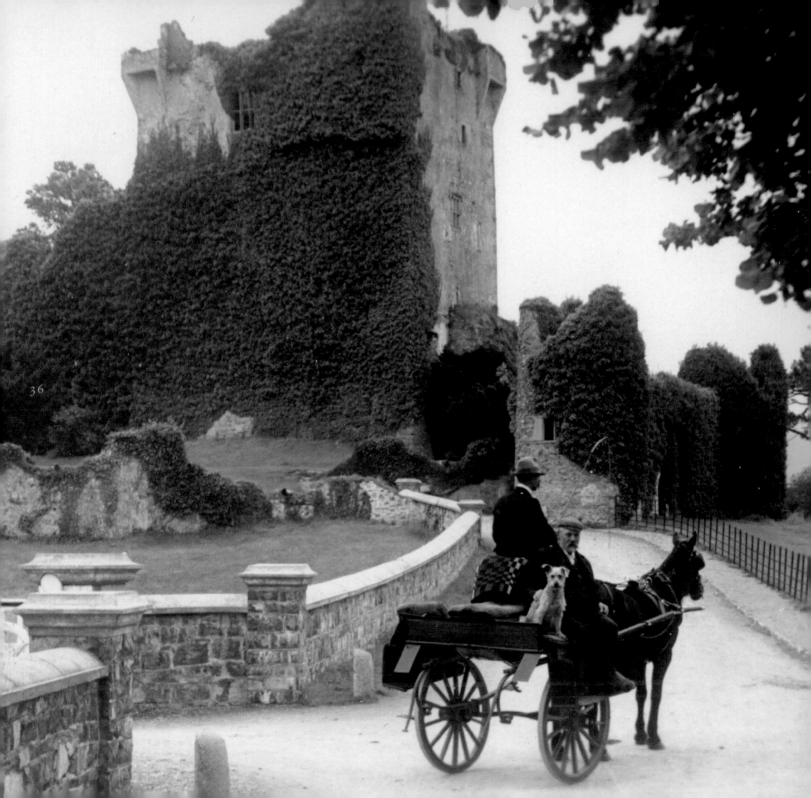

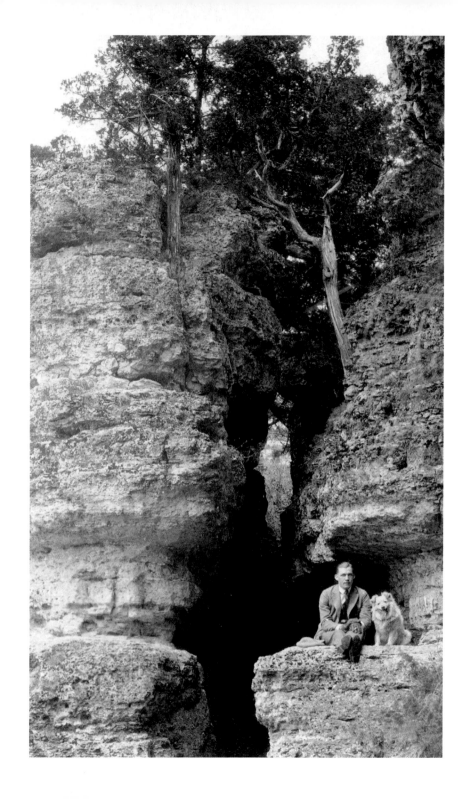

Irish
(opposite)

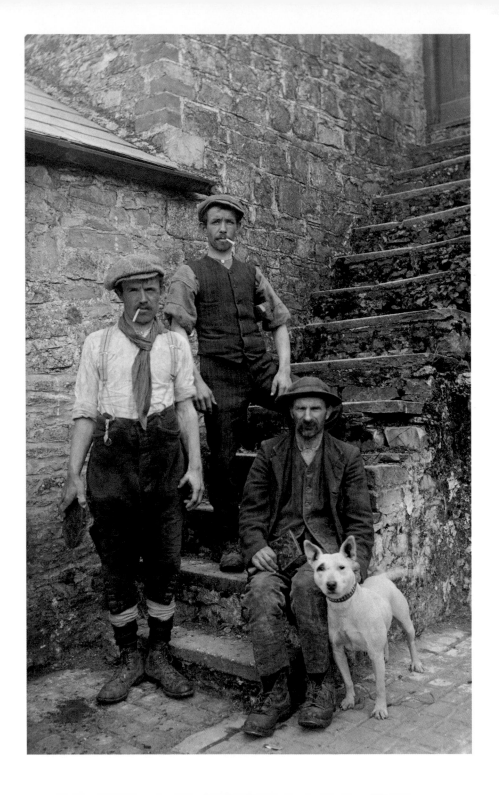

British

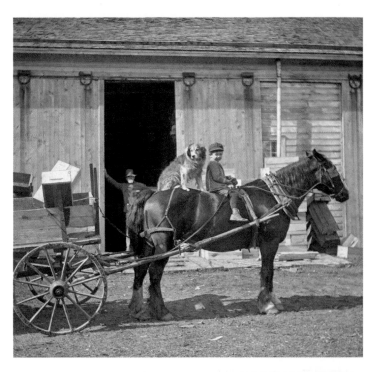

American

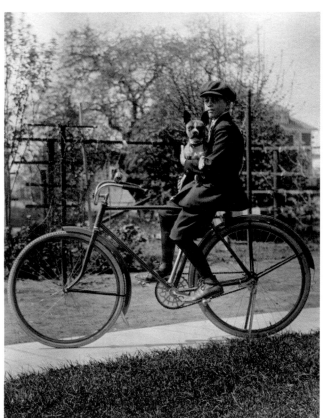

American

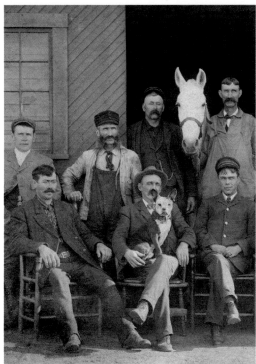

American

Detail from a larger print of railway workers. Printed on reverse are details of the Mt. Washington Railway in New Hampshire.

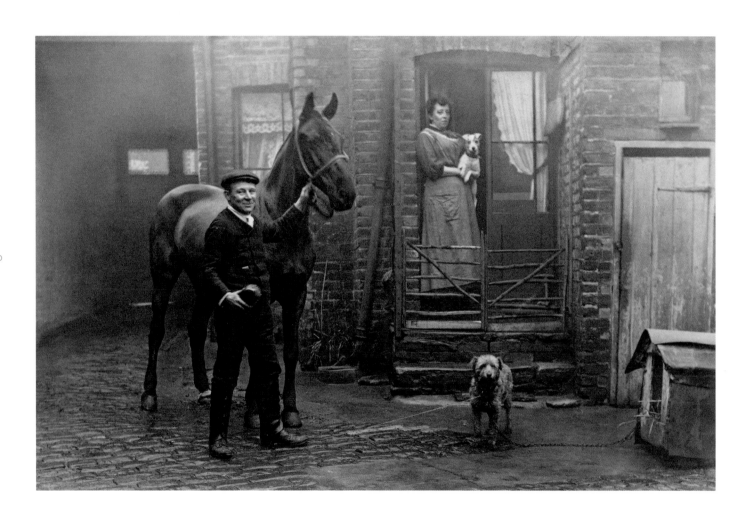

British

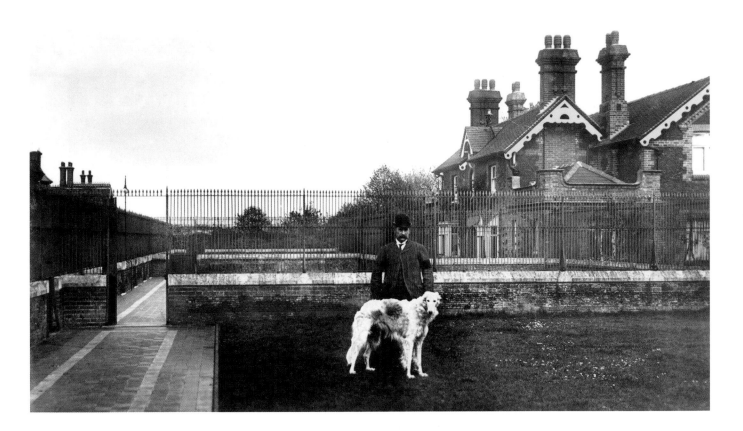

British

The Royal Kennels at Sandringham.
Vassilka, the Queen's favourite
Russian Borzoi.

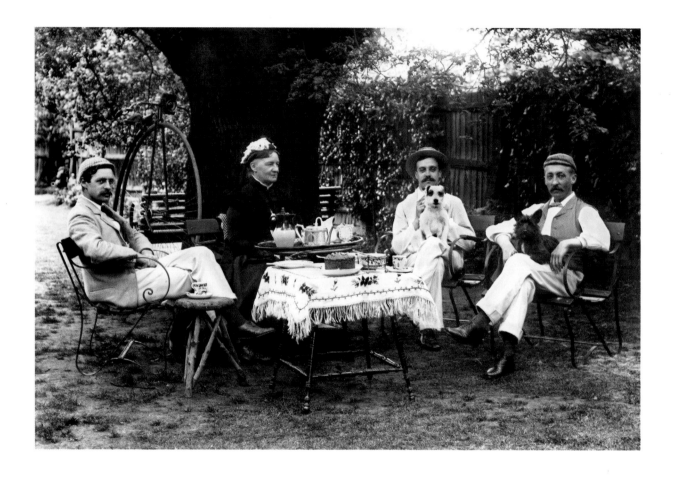

42

British

Notice the penny-farthing leaning against the tree.

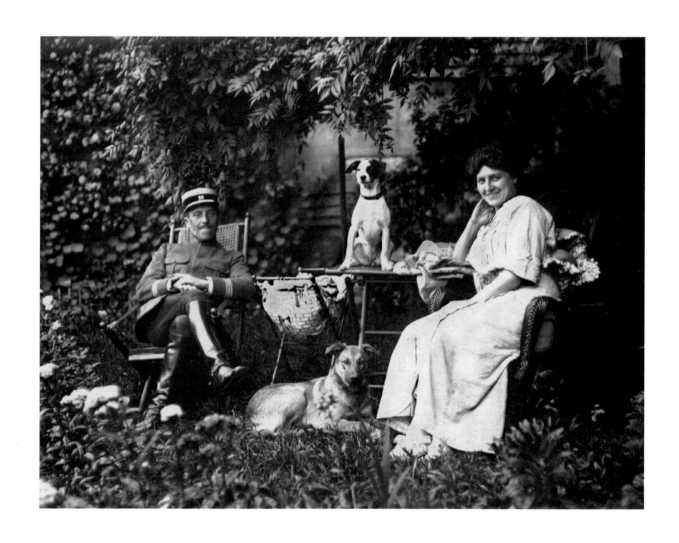

43

44

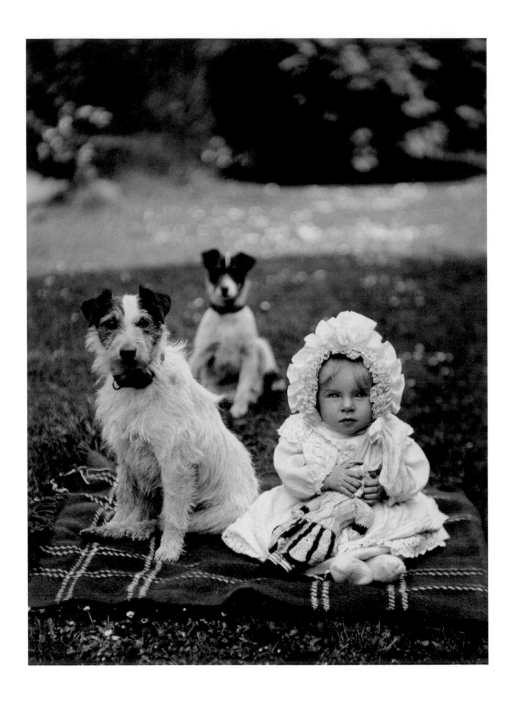

British

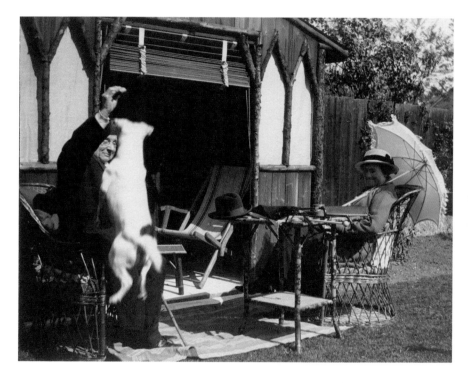

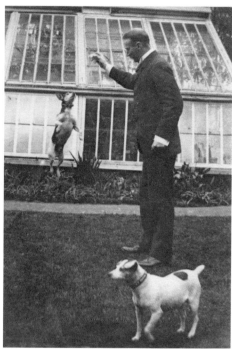

British

Note on reverse: 'Tartar, Bess and Archie April 1894.' In 1894 the fastest shutter speeds were still relatively slow: notice the trail of action from the ground to the leaping dog's bottom paws.

European

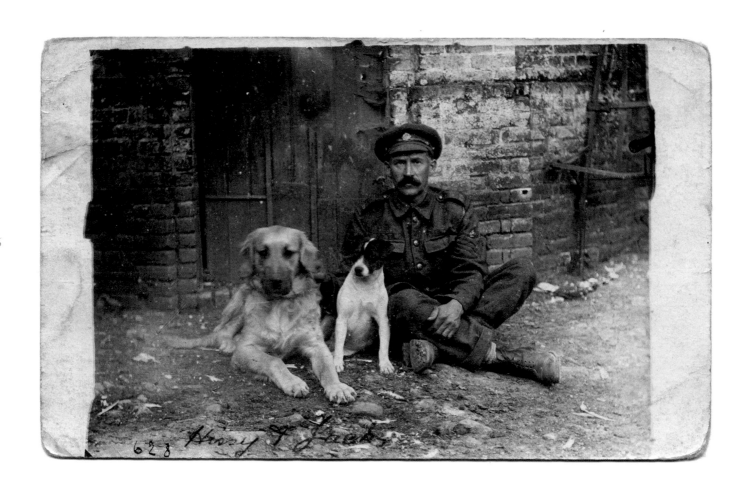

British

Note on reverse: 'France, August 1916.
Our Corp pet. St. Bernard named Hissy
8 months old and the Terrier named
Jack. Just after we came out here 16
months - and our Staff Sgt Farrier
Len Nusse.'

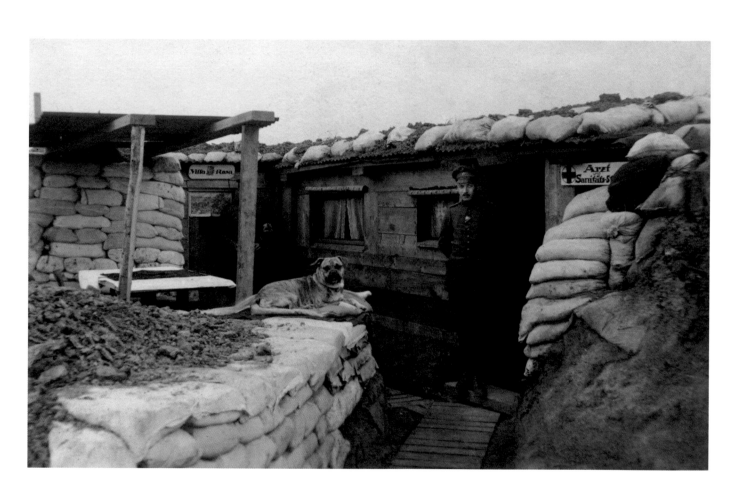

German

Red Cross Station. First World War.

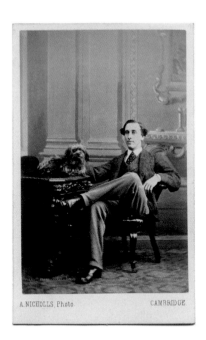

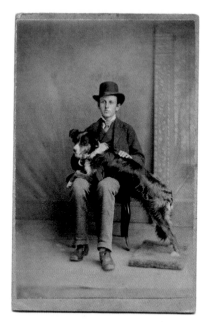

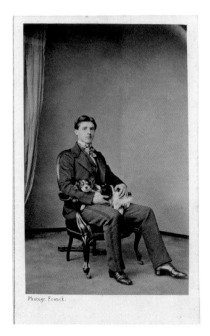

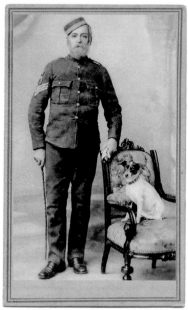

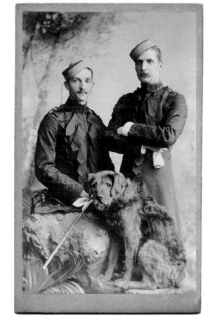

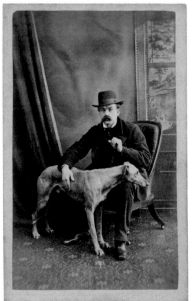

British

British

French. Note on reverse:
'Comte Jean de Colbert'

British

British

British

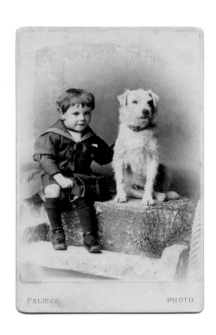

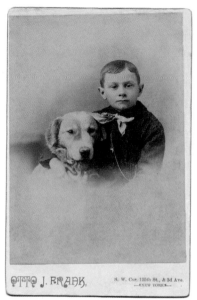

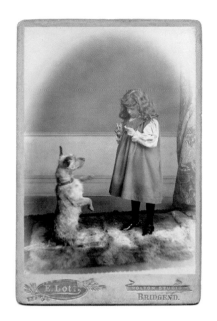

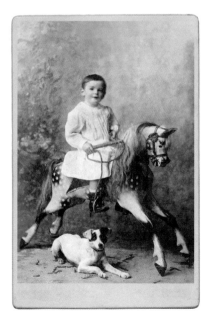

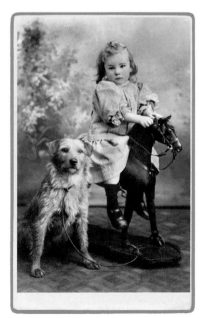

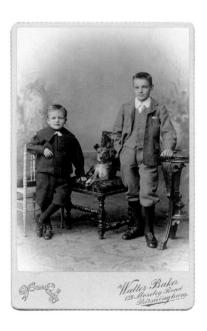

British

British

American

British

British

British

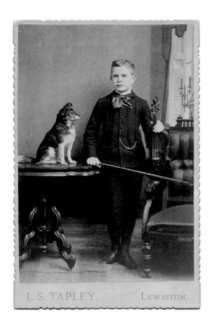

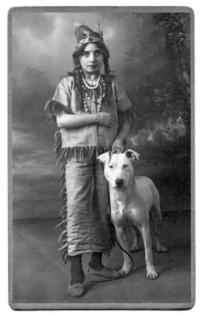

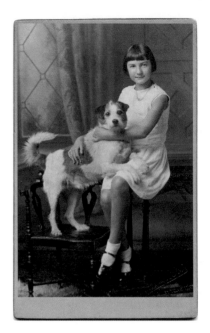

50

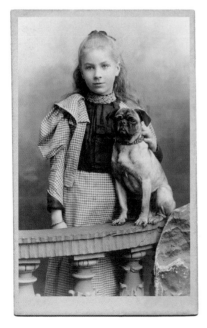

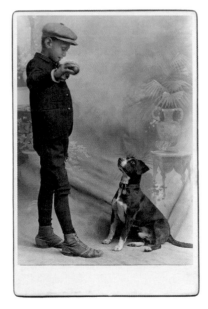

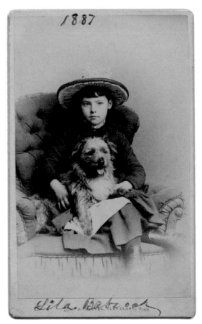

American
British

British
American

British
American

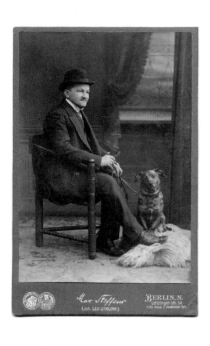

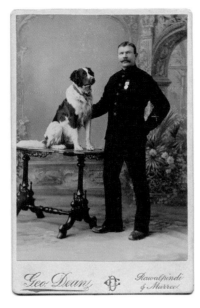

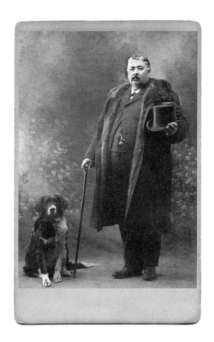

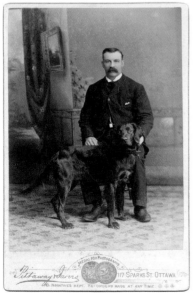

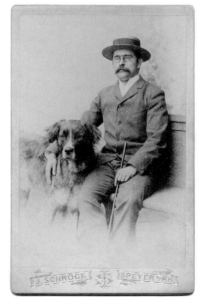

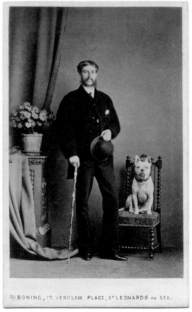

German

Canadian

British in India

German

American

British

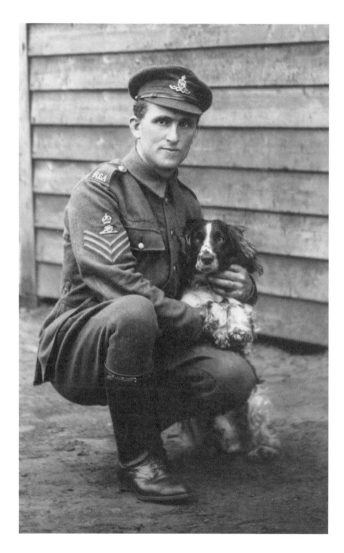

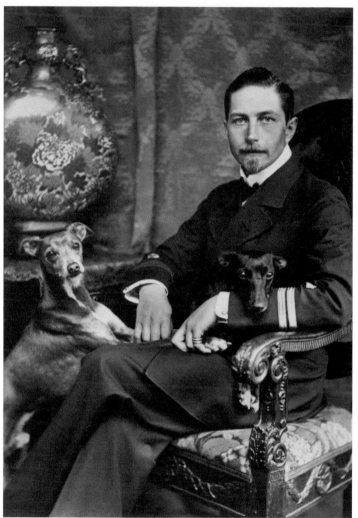

52

British

Prussian

Prinz Adalbert von Preussen.

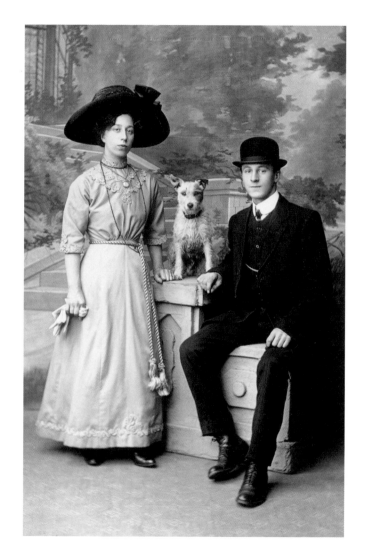

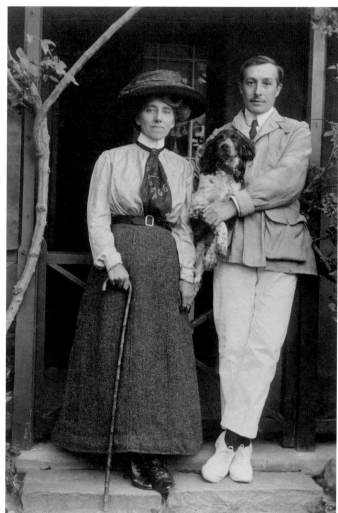

53

British

British

54

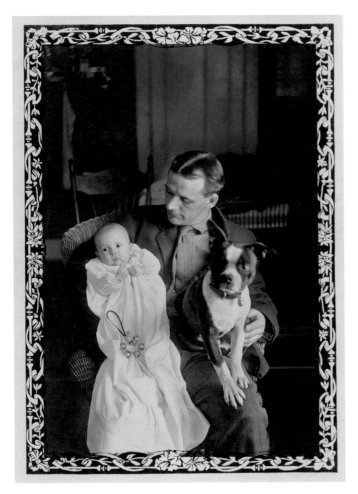

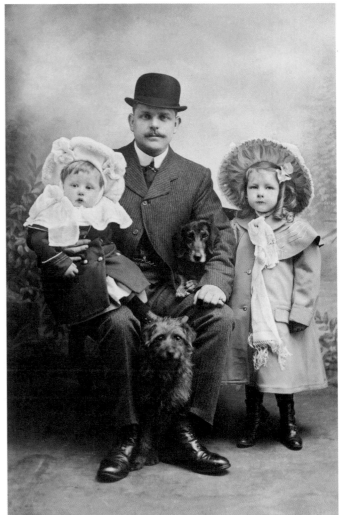

American   British

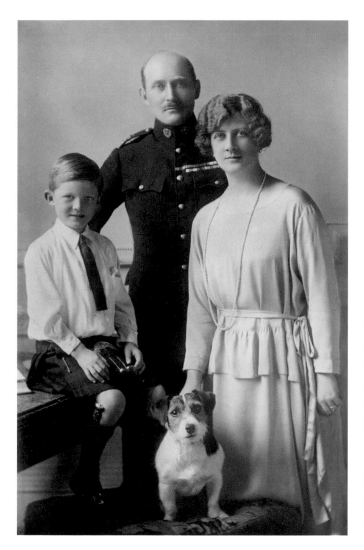

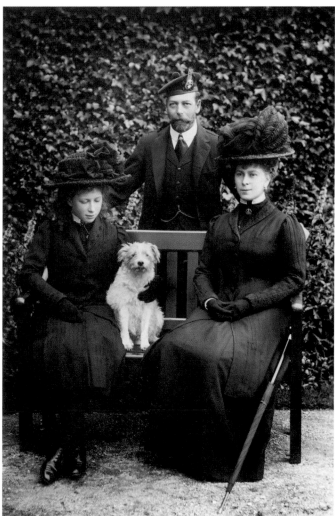

British

Prince Arthur of Connaught and family.

British

Princess Mary, George V and Queen Mary.

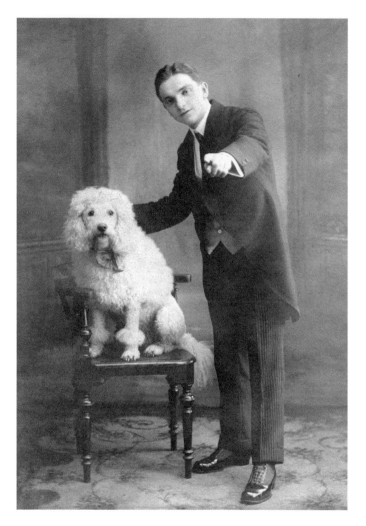

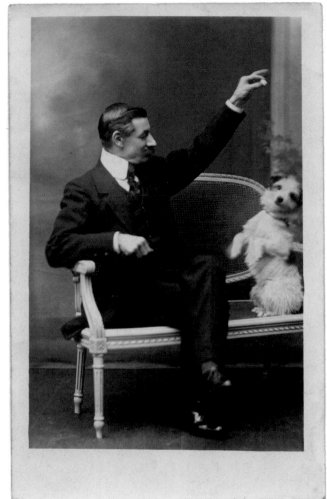

56

Probably European   French

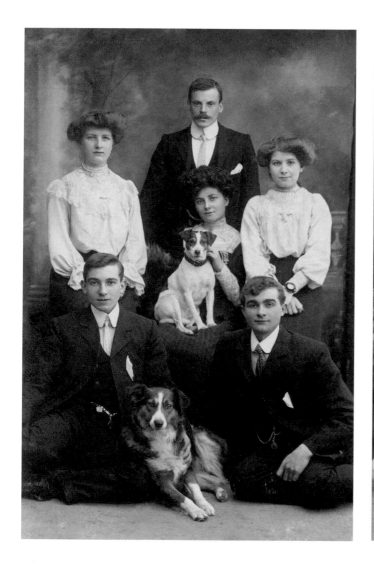

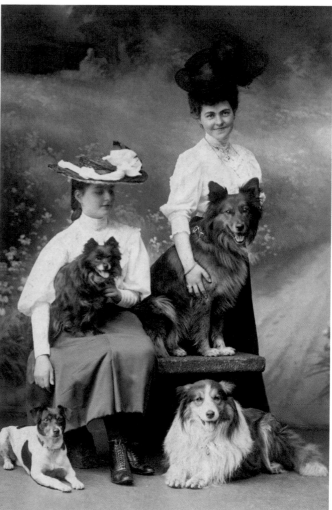

British   German

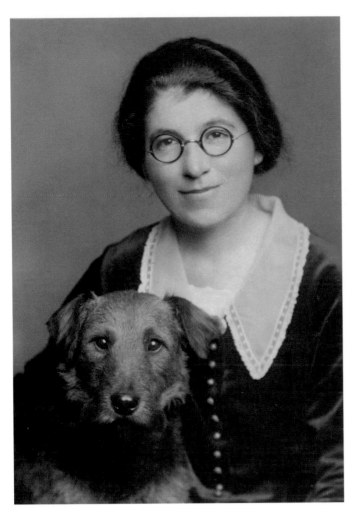

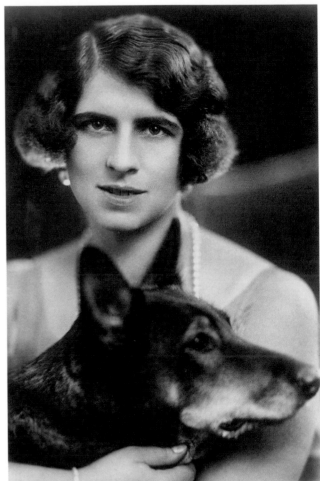

Romanian

Princess Elena of Romania, circa 1923.

British

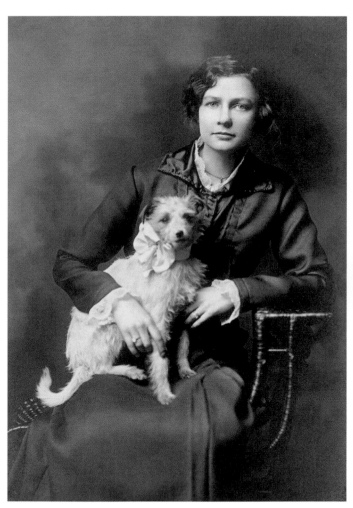

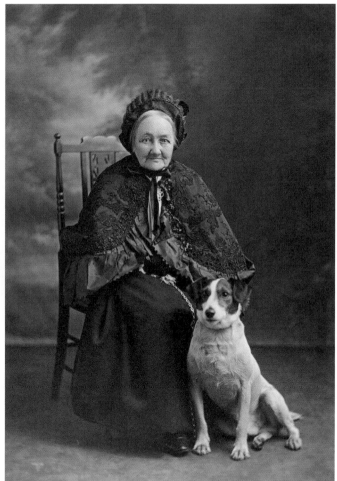

British

British

60

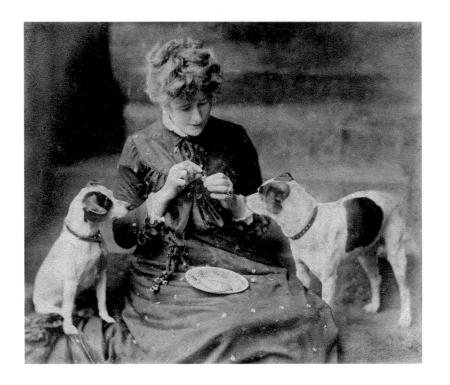

British

Ellen Terry was known for her love of
dogs (as well as for her acting!)

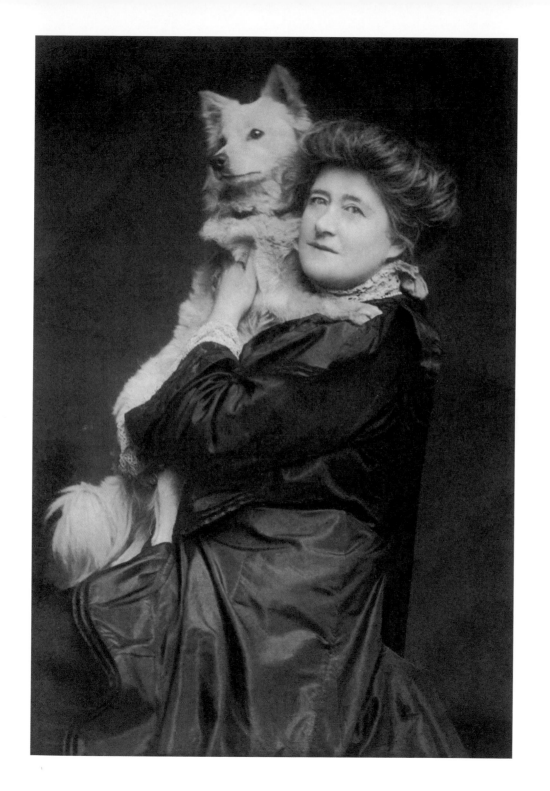

British
Ellen Terry

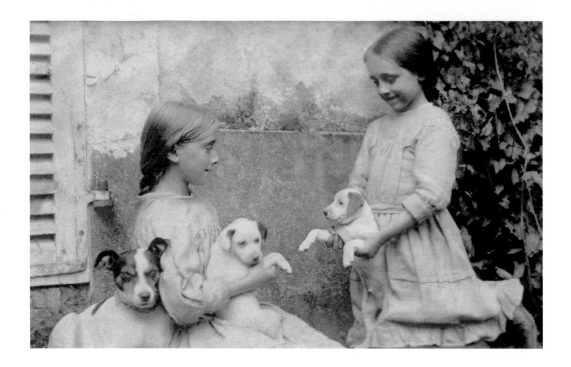

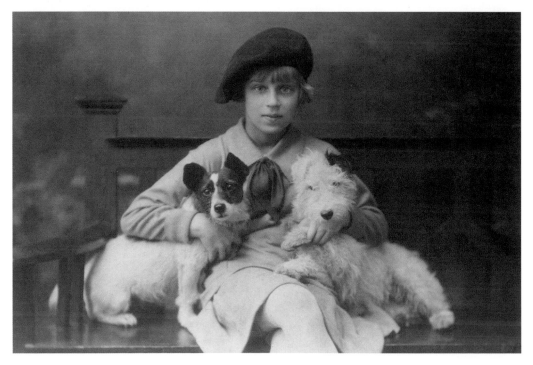

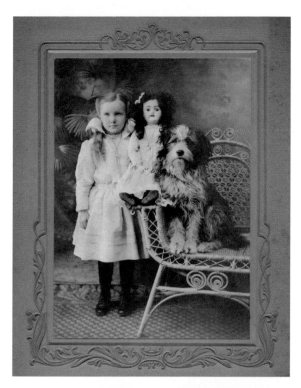

Probably American

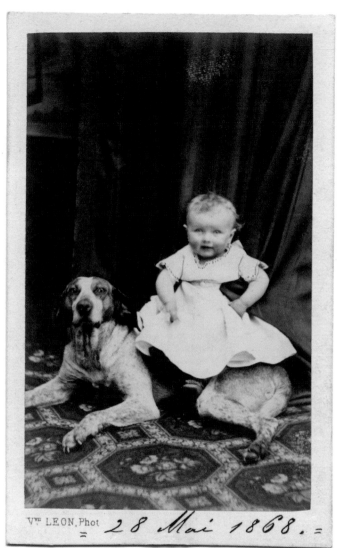

V⁰ LEON, Phot = 28 Mai 1868. =

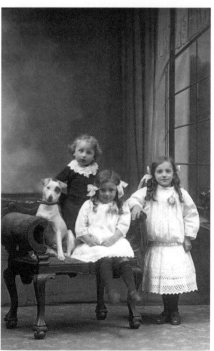

British

French

Notice the hand in the curtain holding the baby!

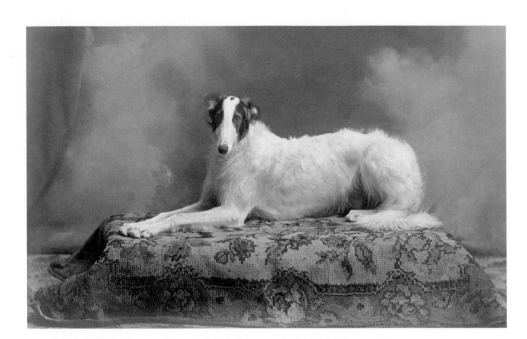

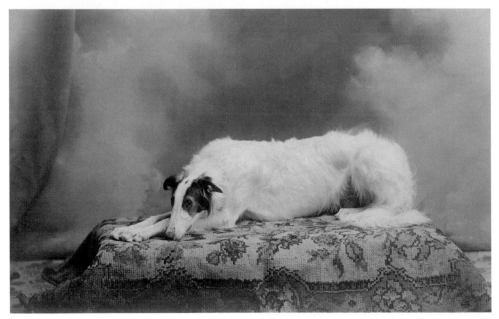

French

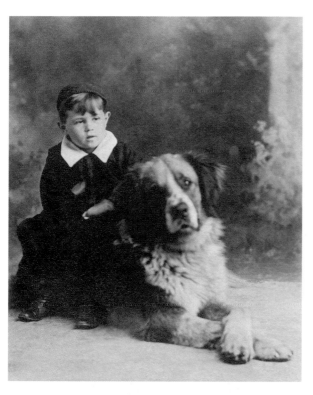

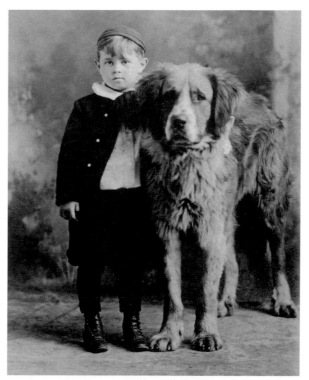

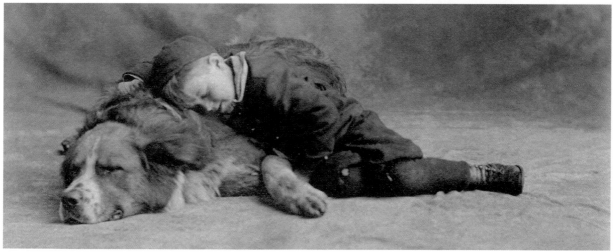

American

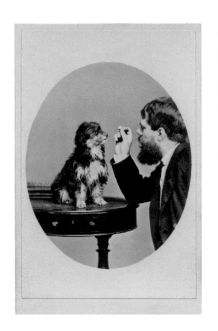

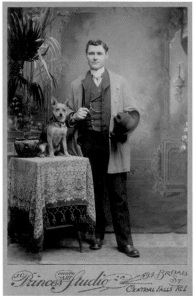

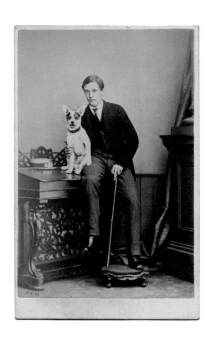

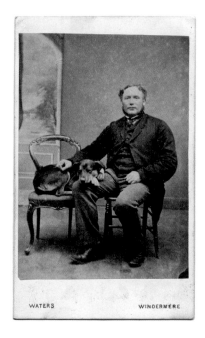

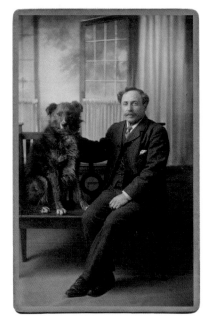

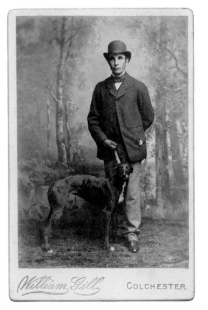

British

American

British

British

British

British

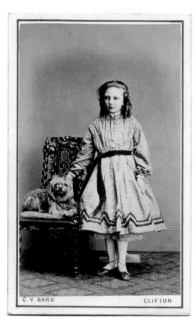
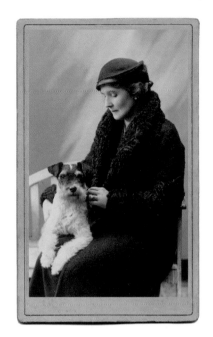
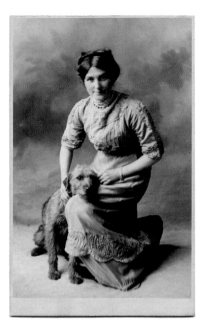

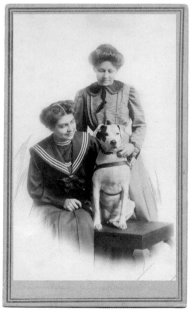
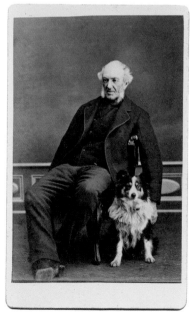
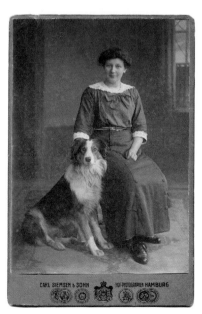

British
American

American
British

British
German

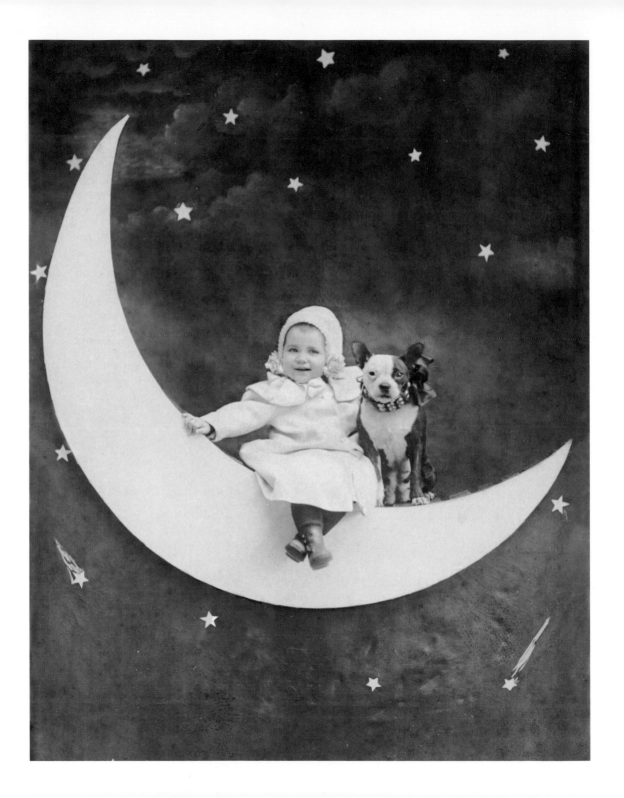

American

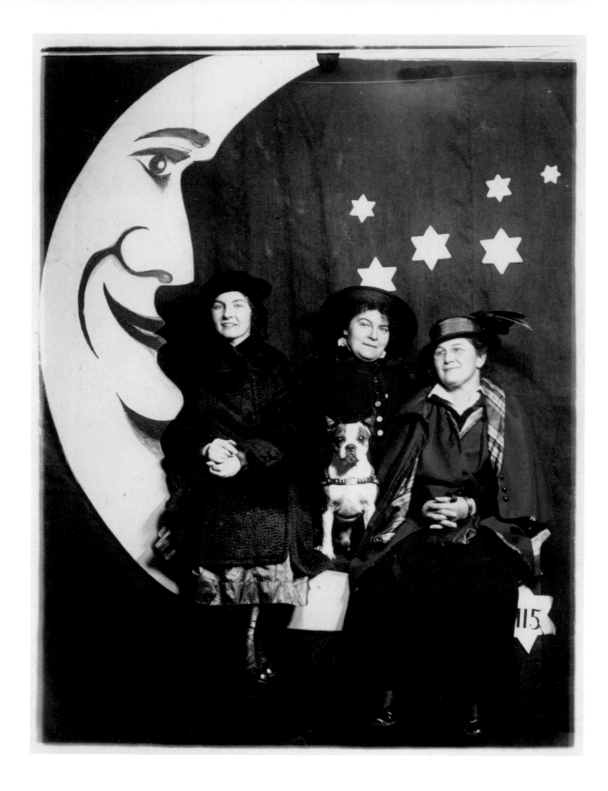

American

On postcard stock.
Note on reverse:
'Was terribly late
getting out to
church. If you
are starving cook
yourself some
boiled ham &
eggs or anything
else you can find.
(Mush or pancakes
in cupboard.)
Otherwise I will be
back at 12:15.'

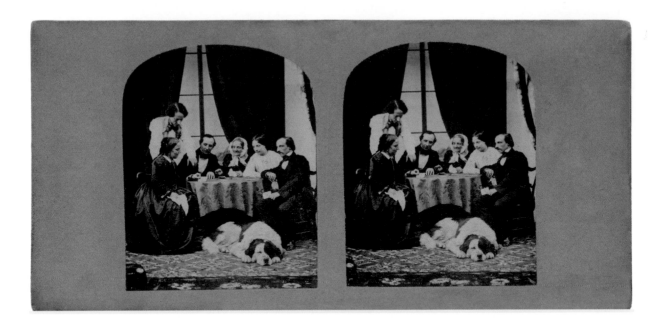

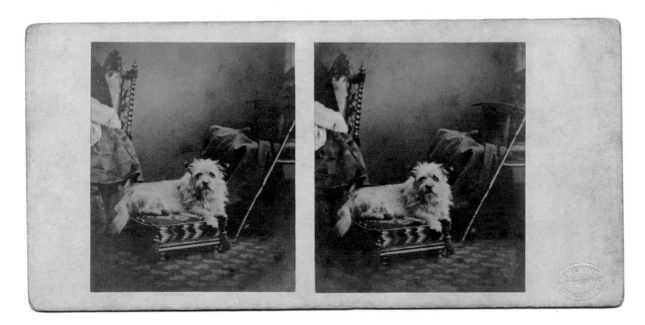

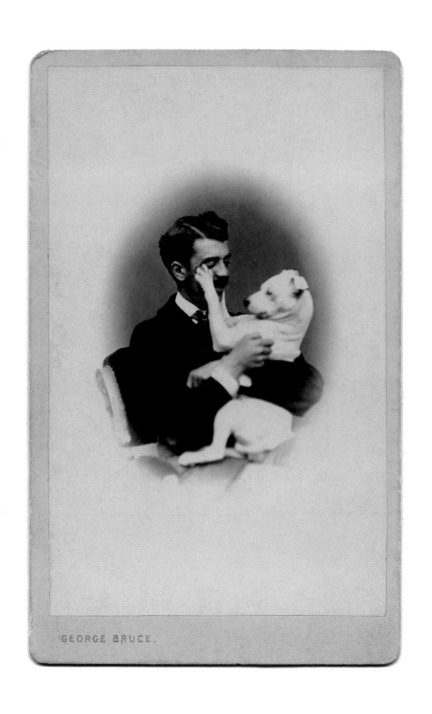

GEORGE BRUCE.

71

Canadian

From album with
note underneath:
'George Home:
(son of the 11th
Earl of Home)'

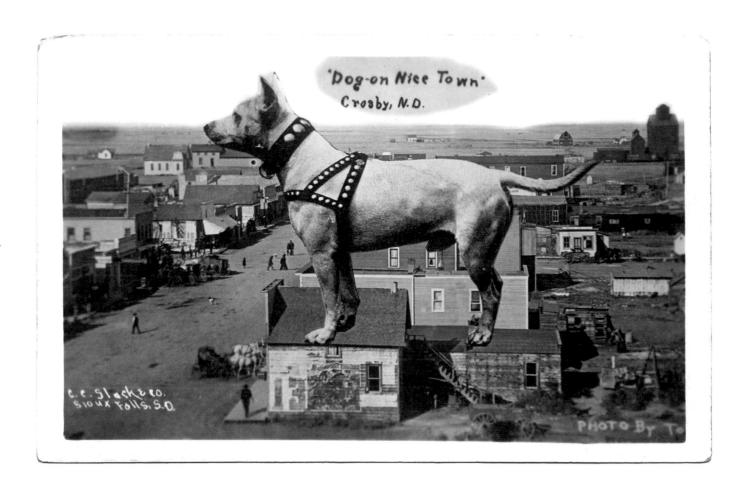

"Dog-on Nice Town"
Crosby, N.D.

C.C. Slack & Co.
Sioux Falls, S.D.

PHOTO BY T.

American

73

Probably German

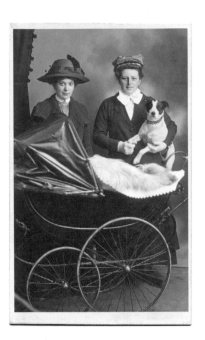

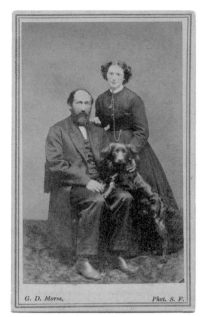

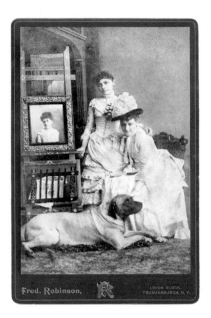

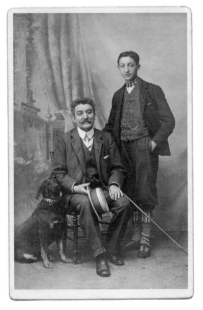

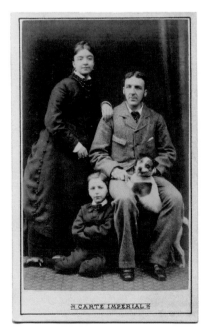

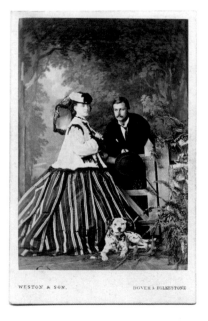

British

French

American

British

American

British

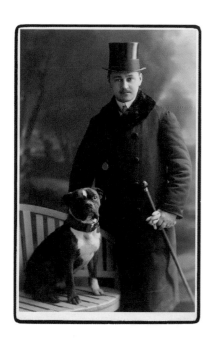
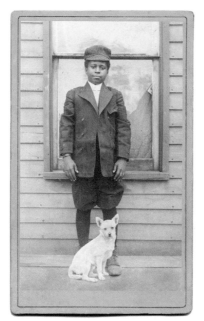
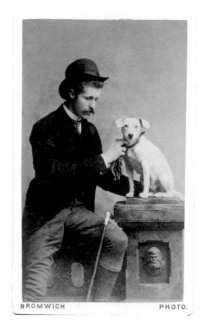

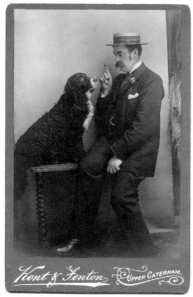
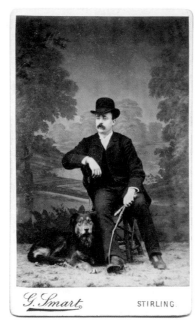
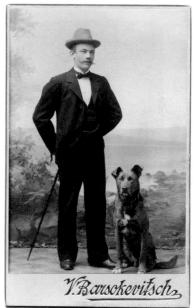

Austrian

British

American

British

British

Finnish

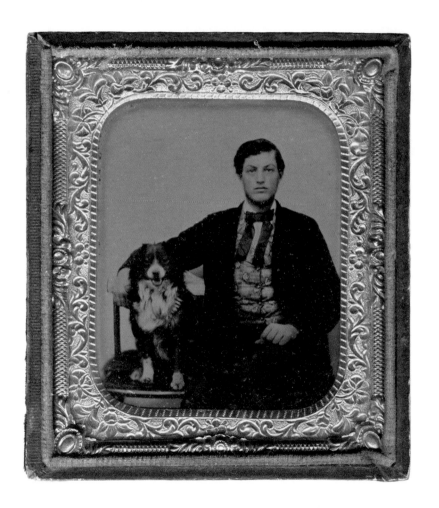

American ambrotype

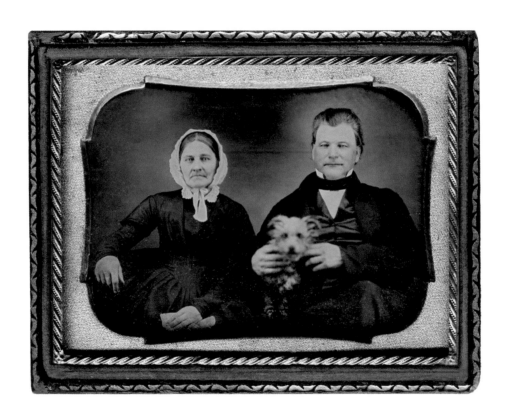

American daguerreotype

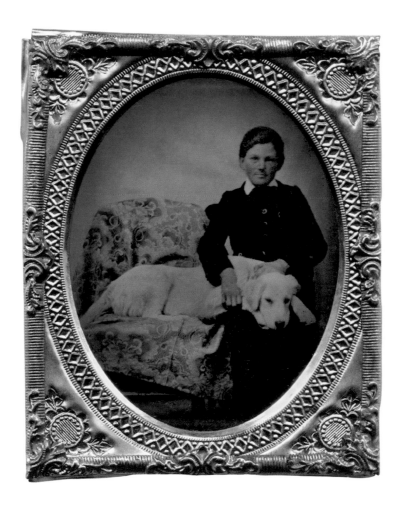

American ambrotype

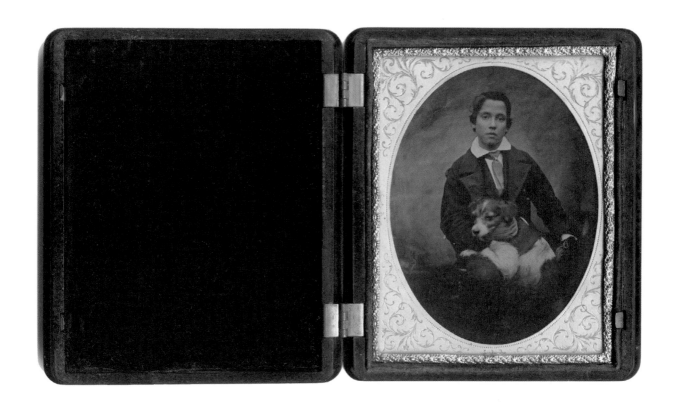

British Quarter-plate ambrotype

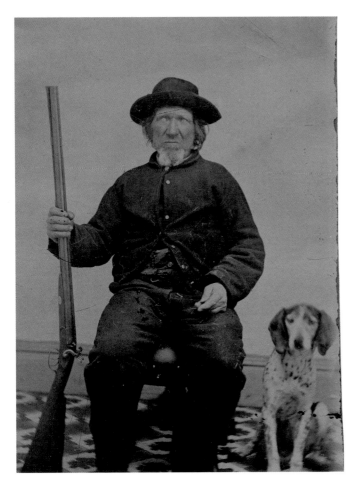

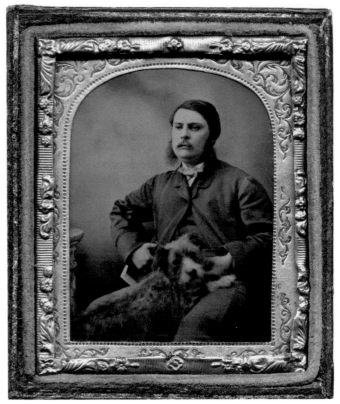

American tintype

American ambrotype

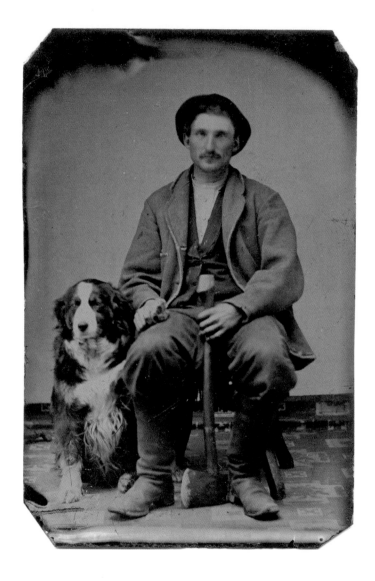

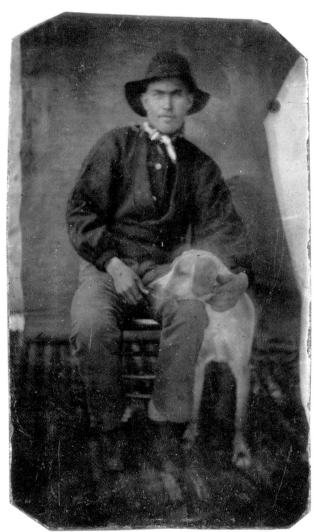

American tintype

American tintype. Probably Kentucky.

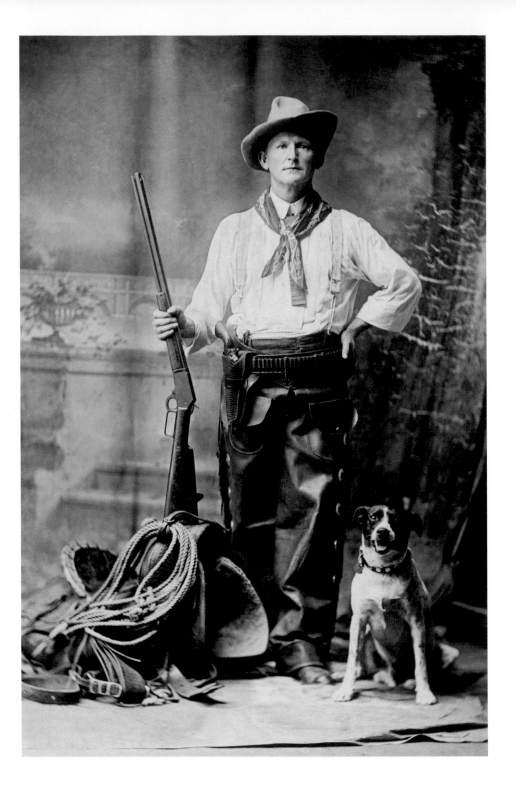

82

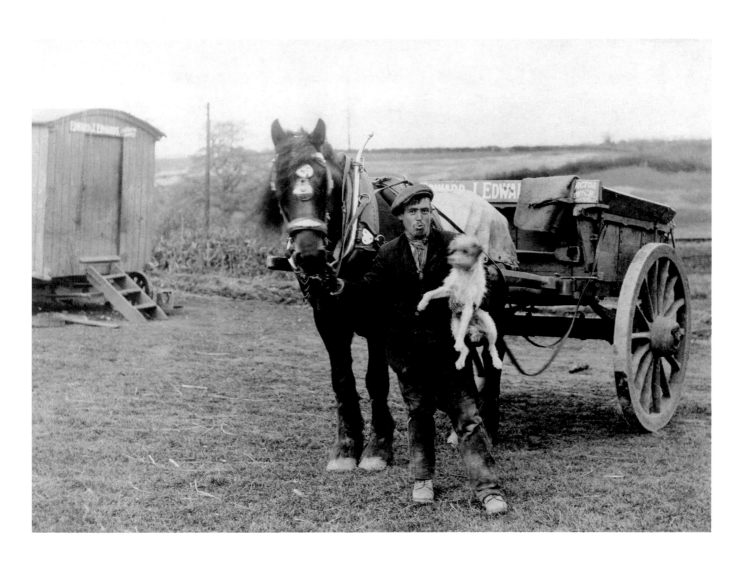

83

British

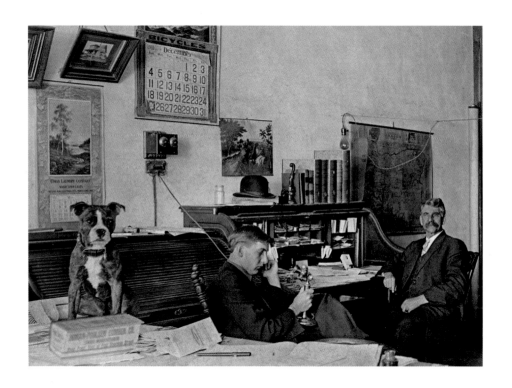

American

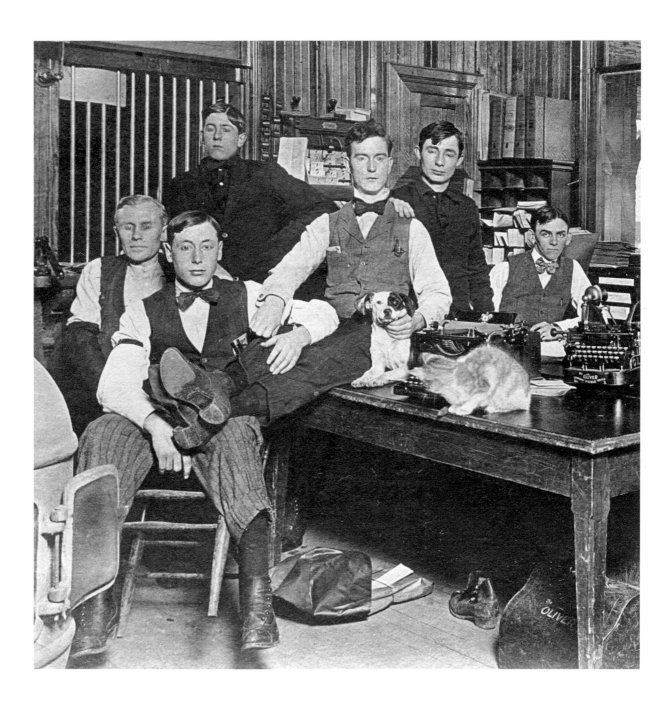

85

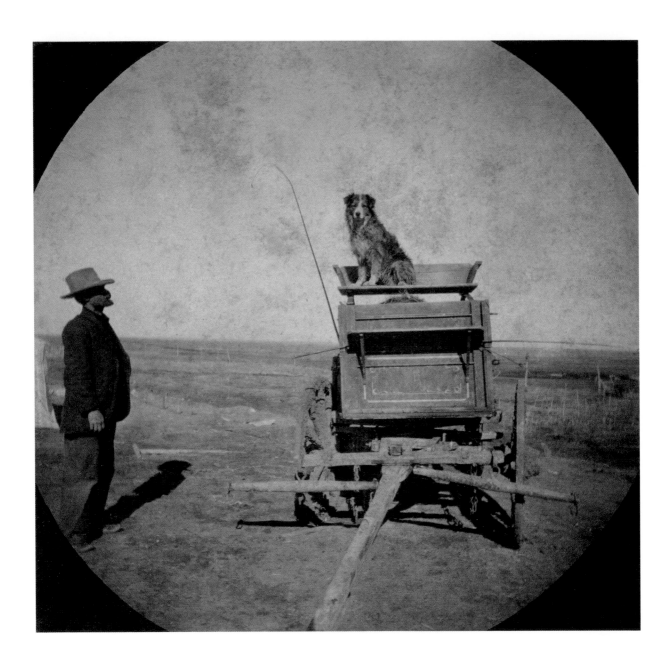

American

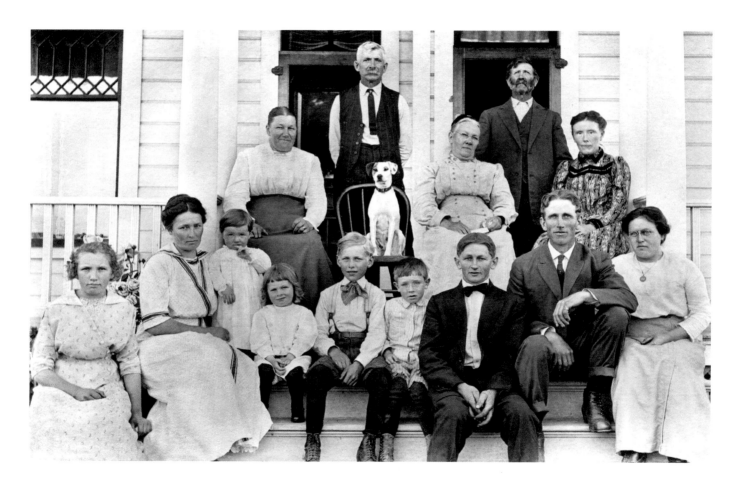

American

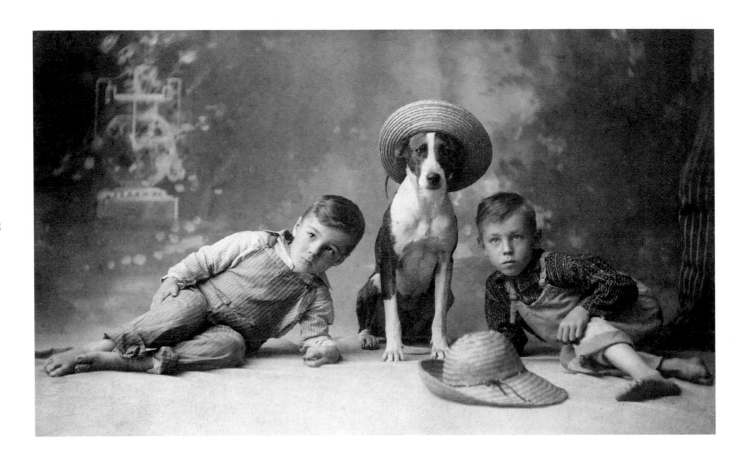

American

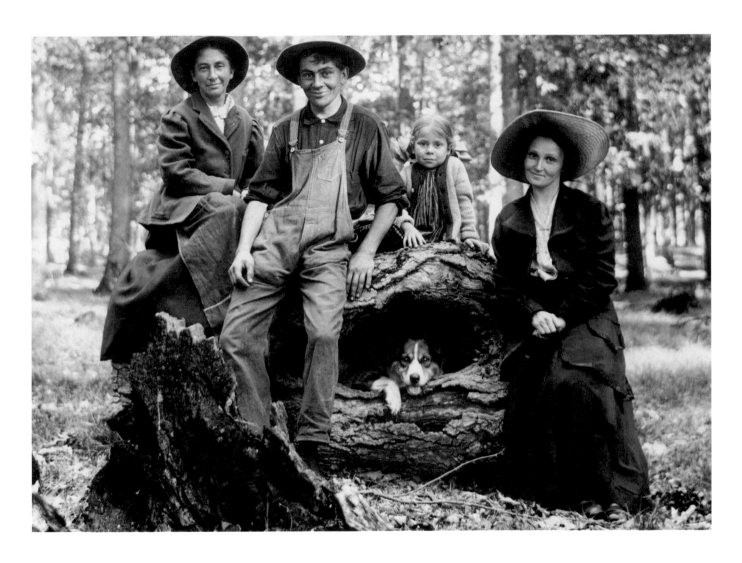

American

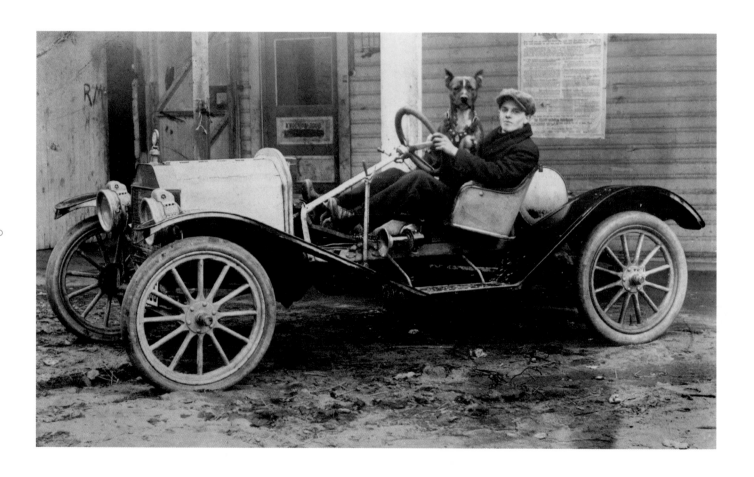

American

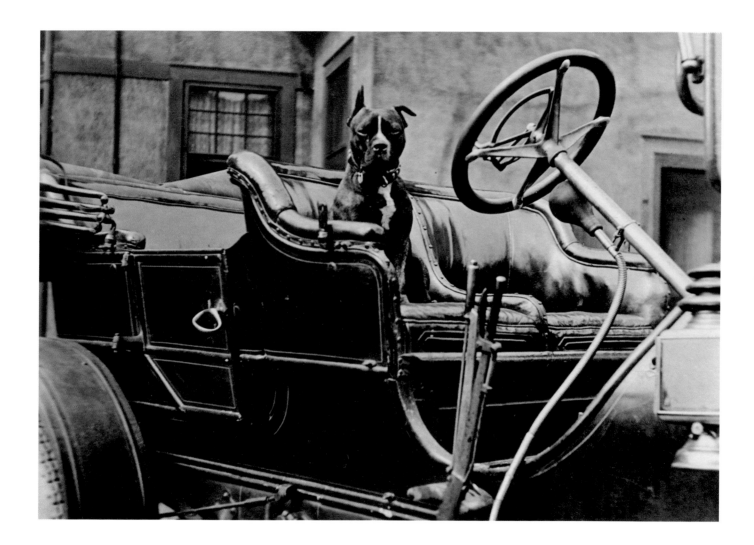

American

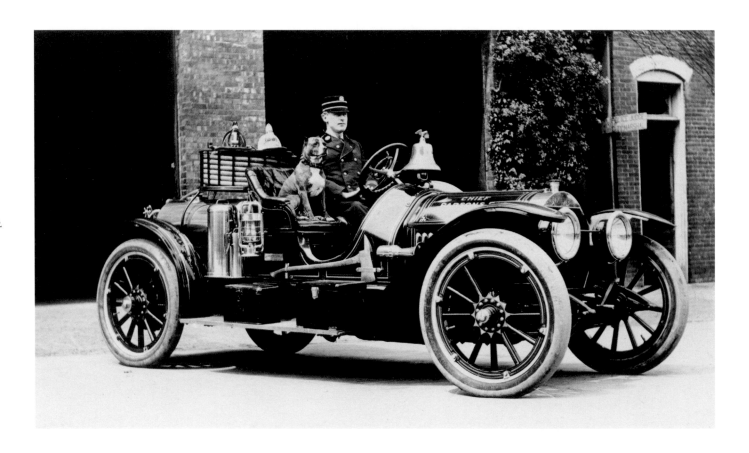

American

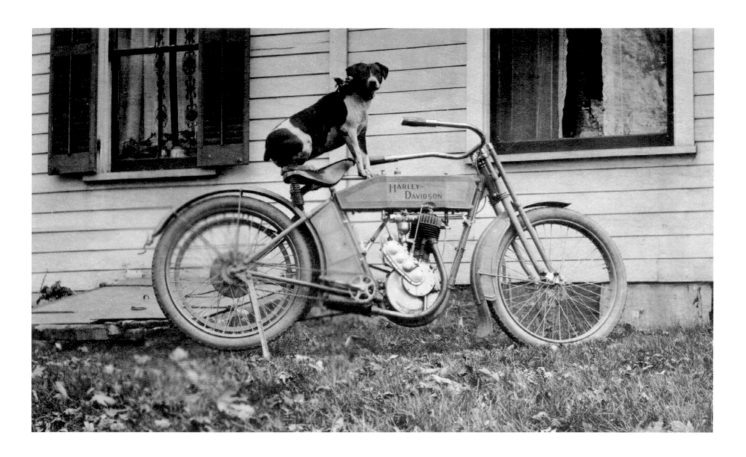

American

94

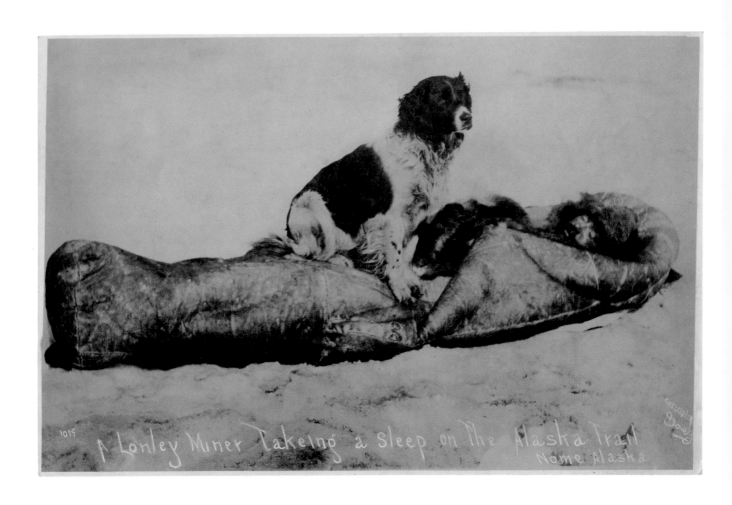

A Lonley Miner Takeing a Sleep on The Alaska Trail
Nome Alaska

American

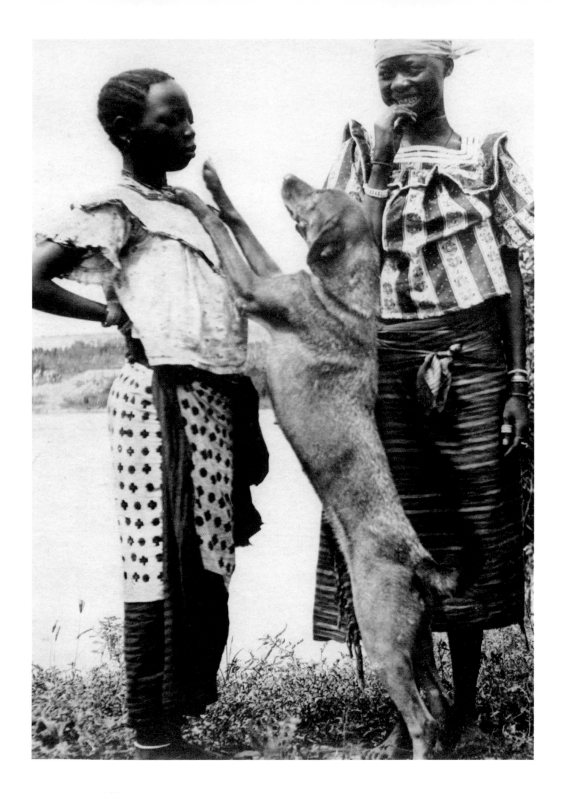

African

Note on reverse:
'Banda, circa 1890'

American

The Yukon. Gold
miners and dog
team north of the
Artic circle, Alaska.

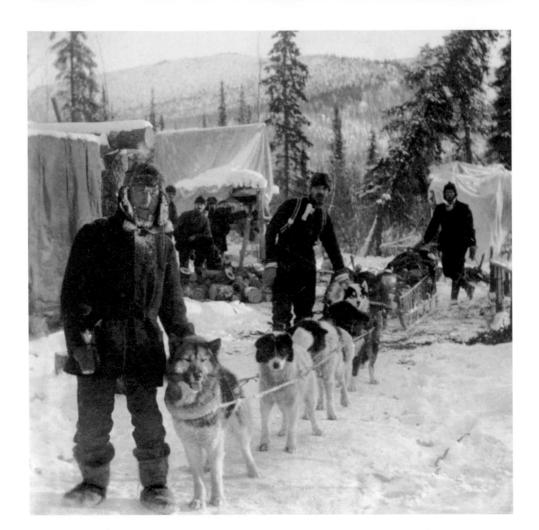

96

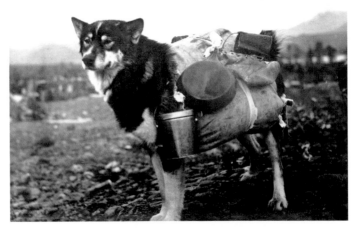

American

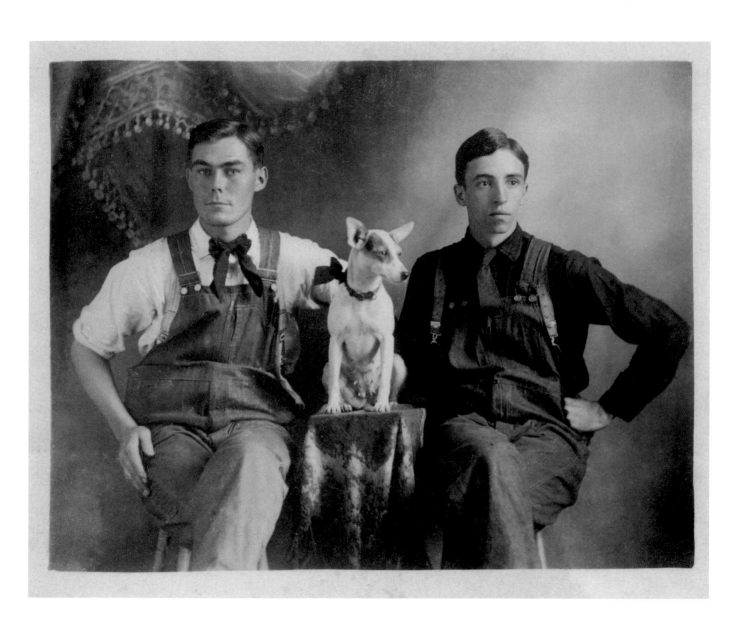

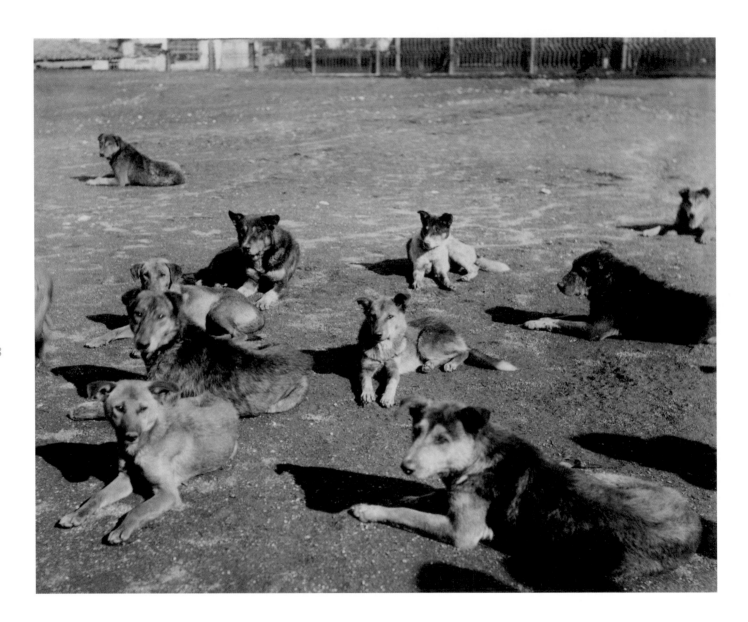

98

Turkish

The famous Dogs of Constantinople, circa 1890. Large unmounted
print by the Gulmez Freres, Constantinople Court photographers.
The Gulmes Freres were three Armenian brothers, Yervant, Kirkor
and Artin Gulmez, who won international prizes for their work
in the 1890s.

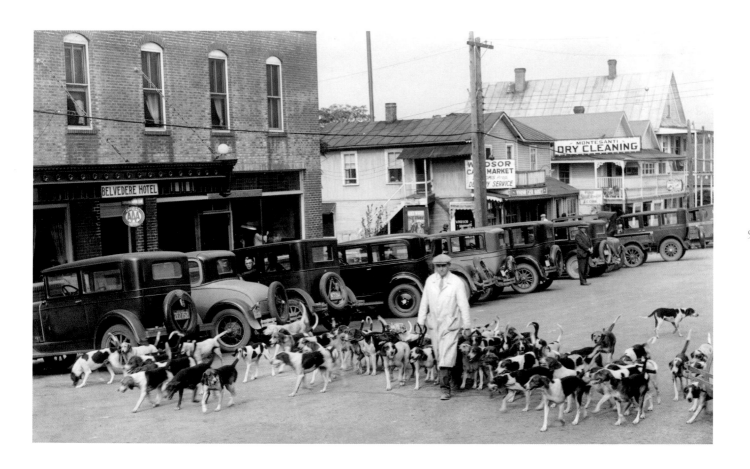

American

Note on reverse: 'Windsor New Jersey.'
Circa 1929.

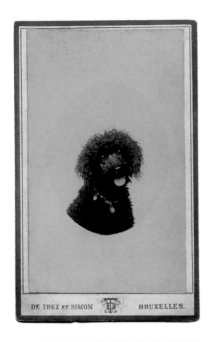

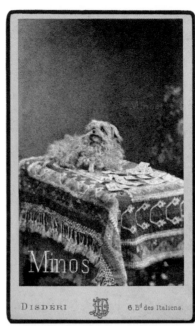

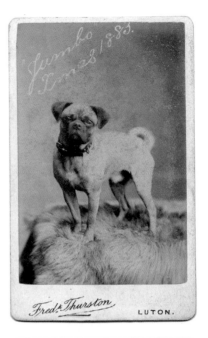

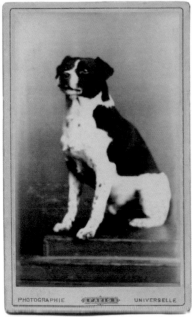

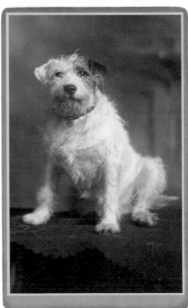

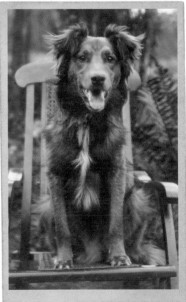

Belgian

French

French. Photograph by Disdéri,
the inventor of the *carte-de-visite*.

British

British

British

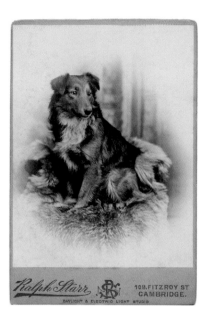

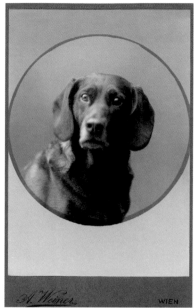

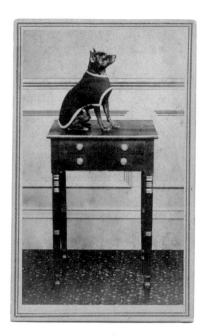

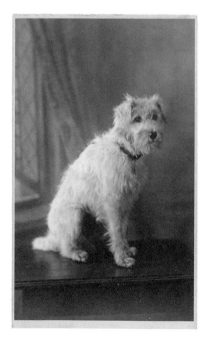

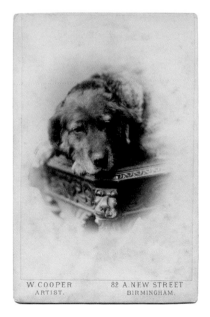

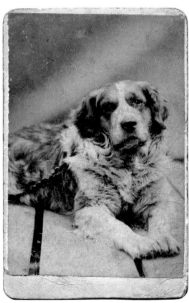

British

British

Austrian

British

British

Probably European

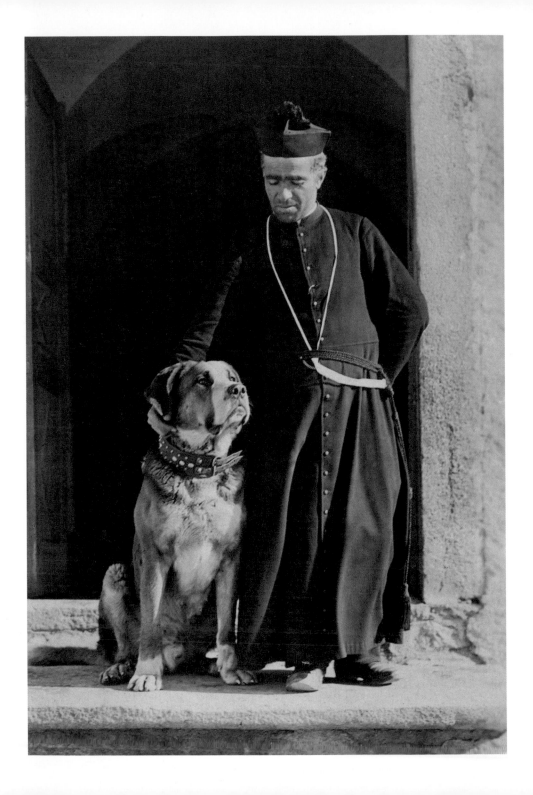

Swiss

Grand St Bernard

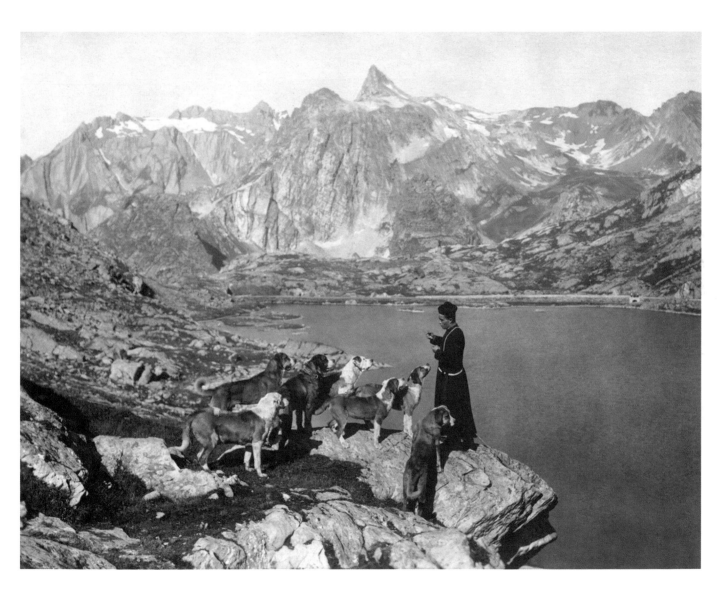

Swiss

Grand St Bernard

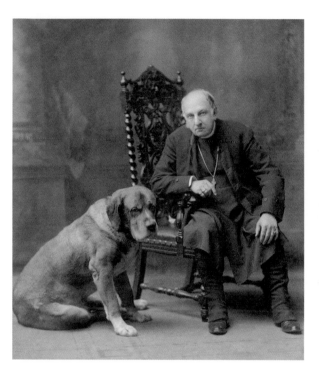

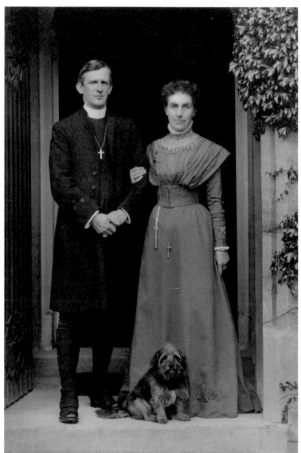

American

British

The Bishop of Lewes & Mrs. Burrows.

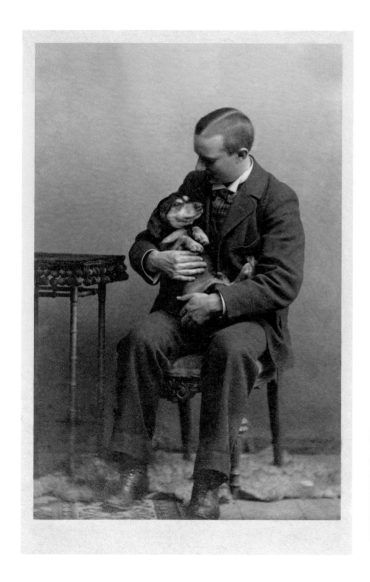

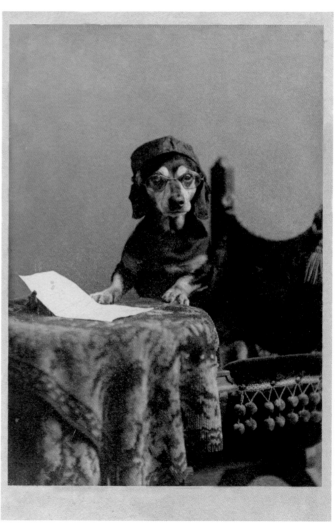

German

German

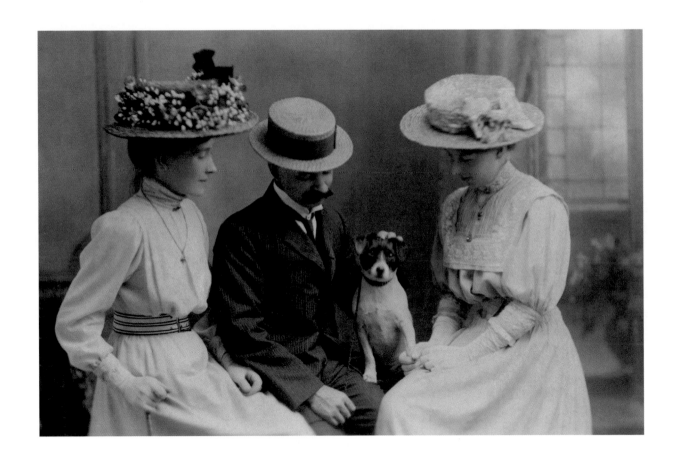

British

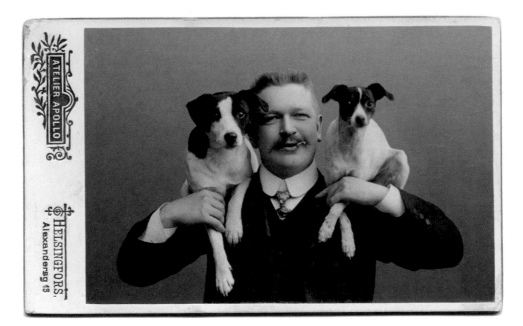

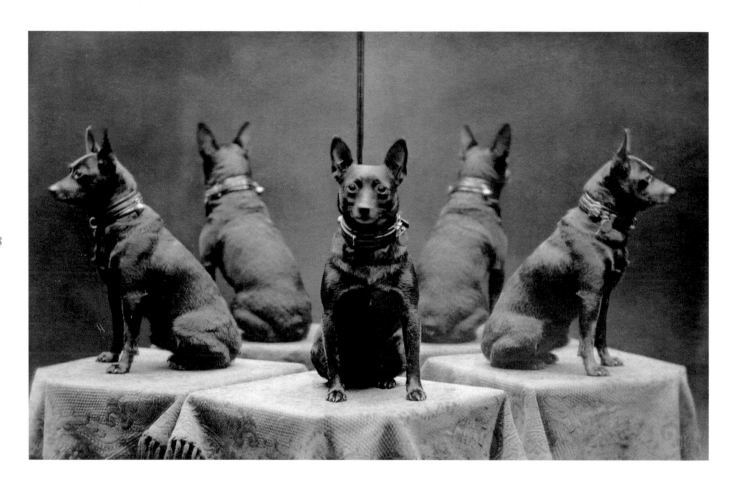

American. Note on reverse: 'boardwalk Atlantic city.'

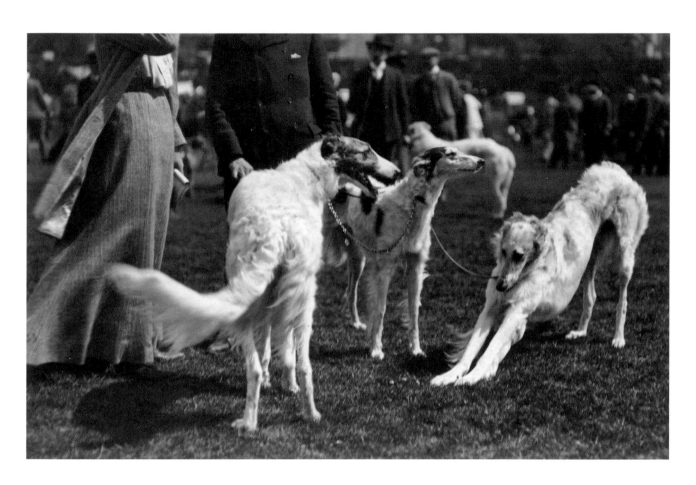

British

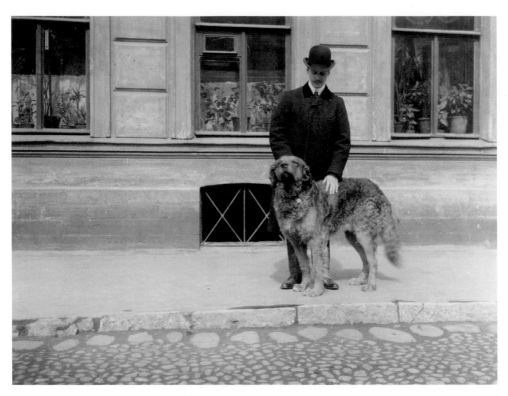

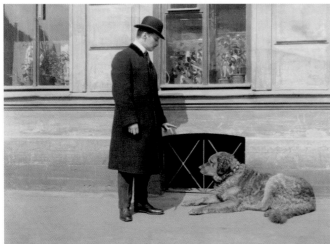

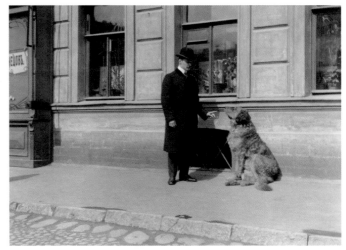

Russian
1906

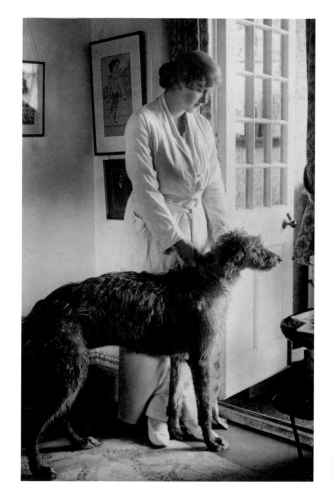

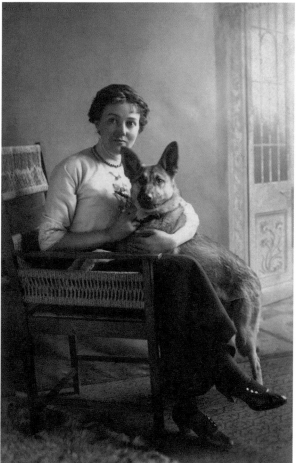

British

The celebrated beauty Gladys Cooper, whose many acting roles included, in later years, Maxim de Winter's sister in the film *Rebecca* and Henry Higgins's mother in *My Fair Lady*.

German

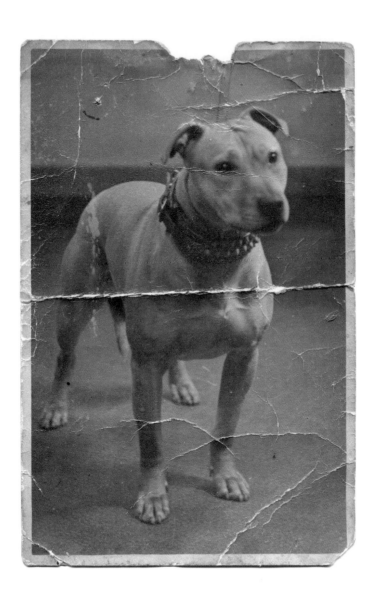

112

British

This photograph,
with the note 'Mick'
on the reverse, had
been kept with
the collar Mick is
wearing.

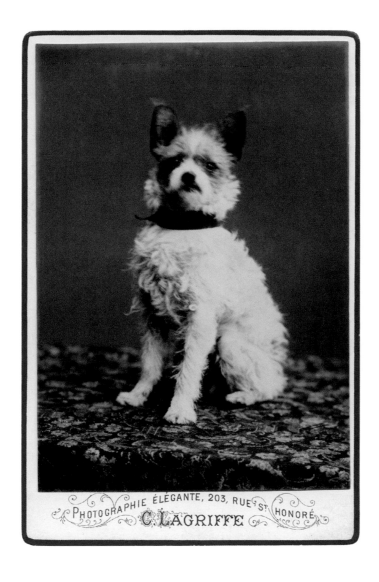

Photographie Élégante, 203, Rue St Honoré
C. LAGRIFFE

French

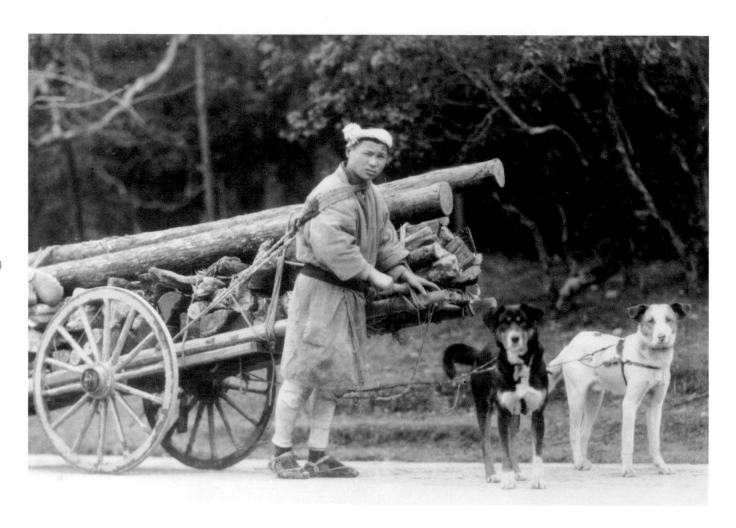

Japanese

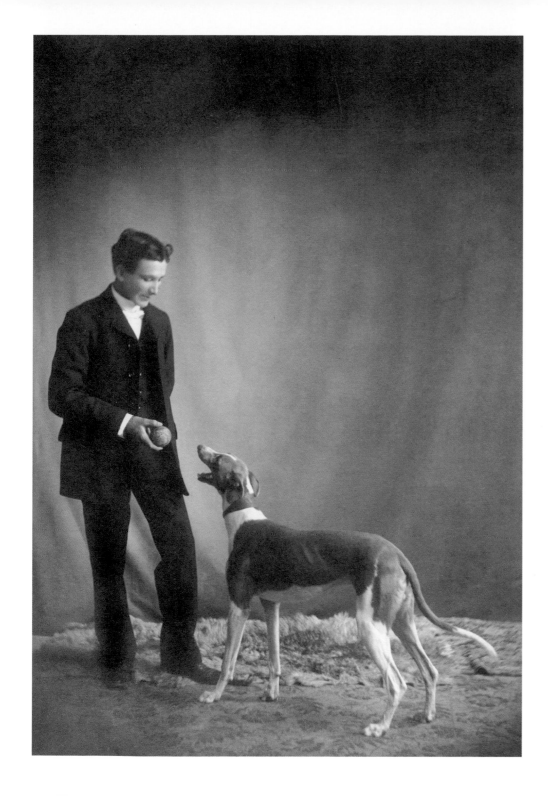

American

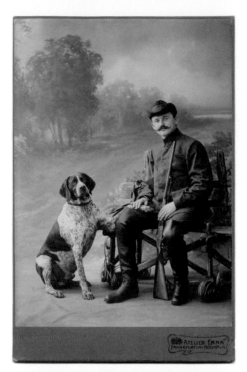

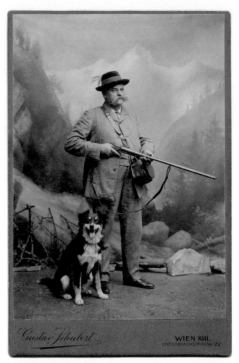

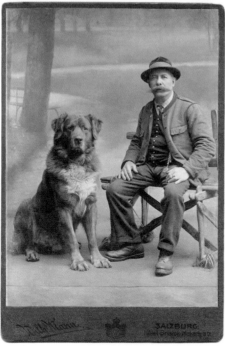

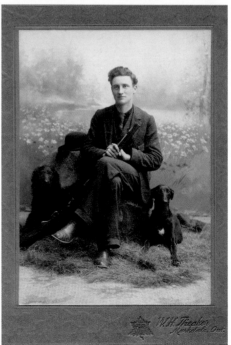

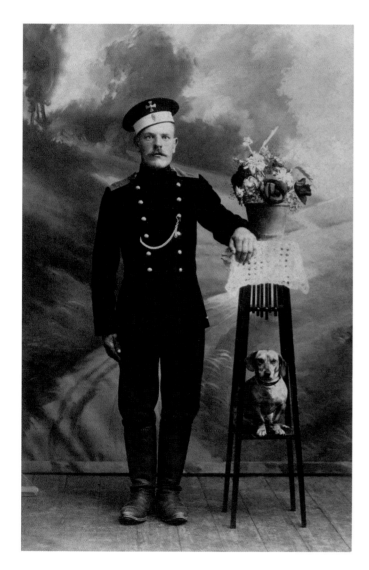

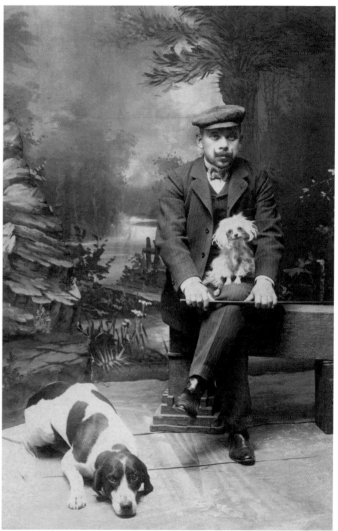

Russian

European

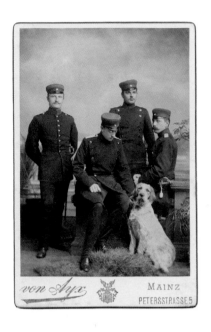

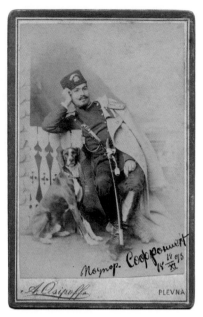

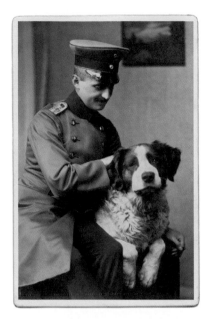

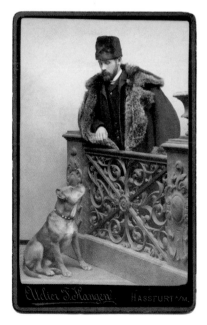

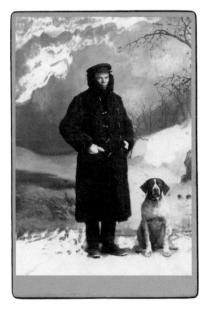

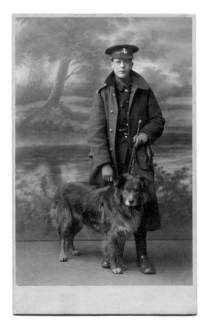

German

German

Bulgarian

Canadian, circa 1918

German

British

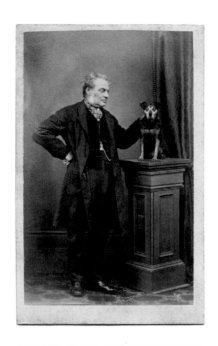

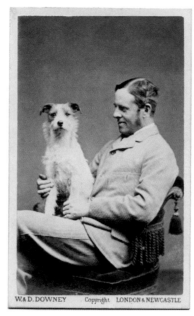

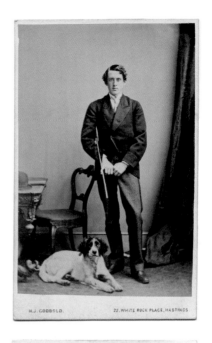

W.& D. DOWNEY   Copyright   LONDON & NEWCASTLE

H.J. COBBOLD.   22. WHITE ROCK PLACE, HASTINGS.

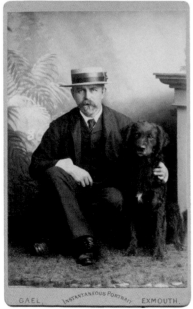

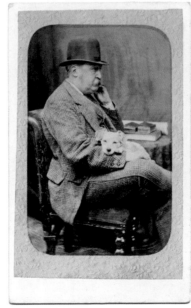

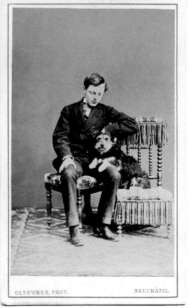

GAEL.   INSTANTANEOUS PORTRAIT   EXMOUTH.

OLSOMMER. PHOT.   NEUCHÂTEL.

British

British

British

British

British

British

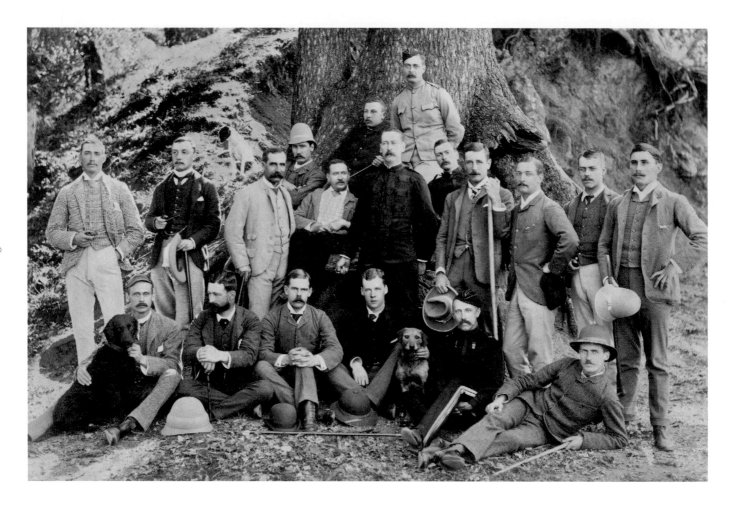

British in India

Changla Gali: Indian Army School of Musketry,
near the hill station of Muree.
(Spot the third dog!)

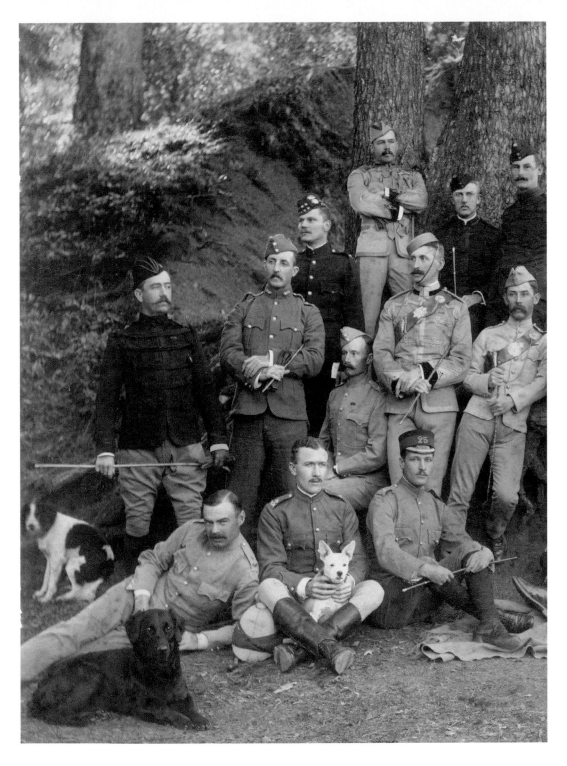

British in India

Detail from a second
photograph of the School
of Musketry. Perhaps some
of these are the same men
and dogs as in the previous
photograph?

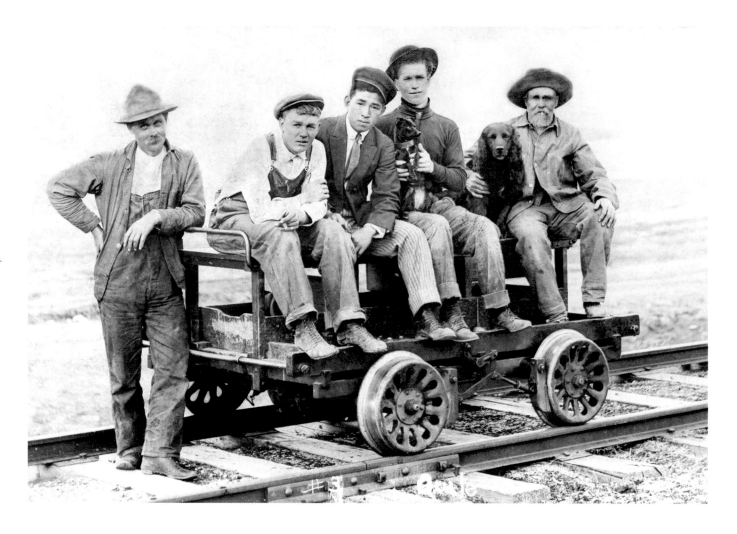

American

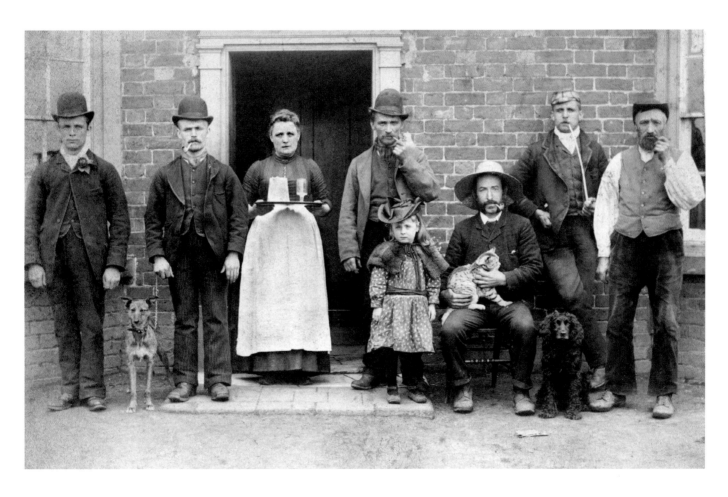

British

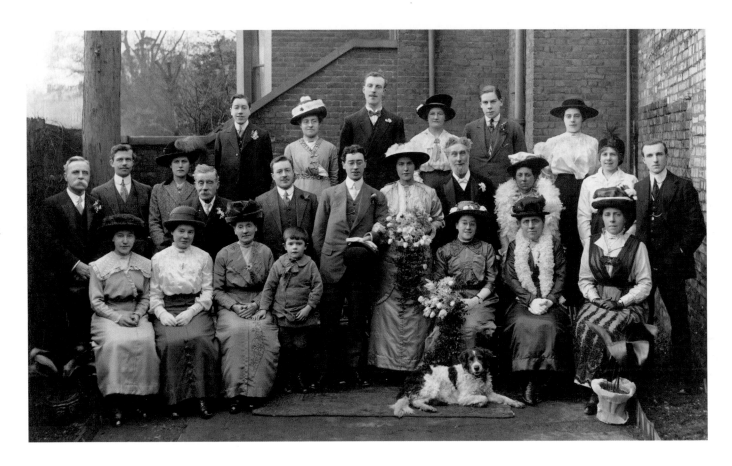

British

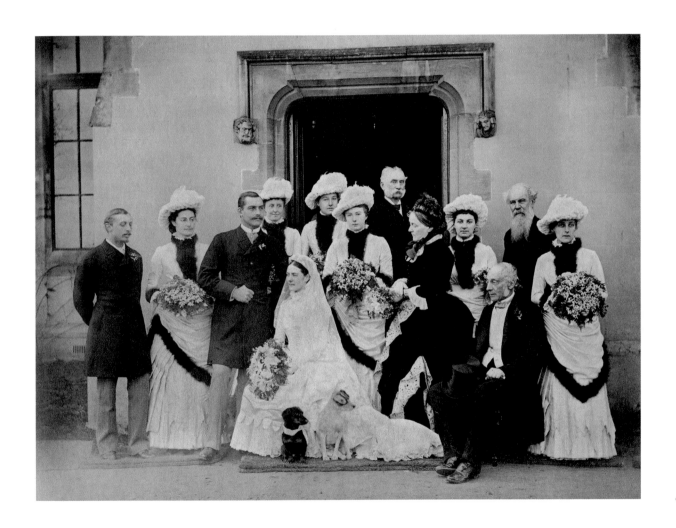

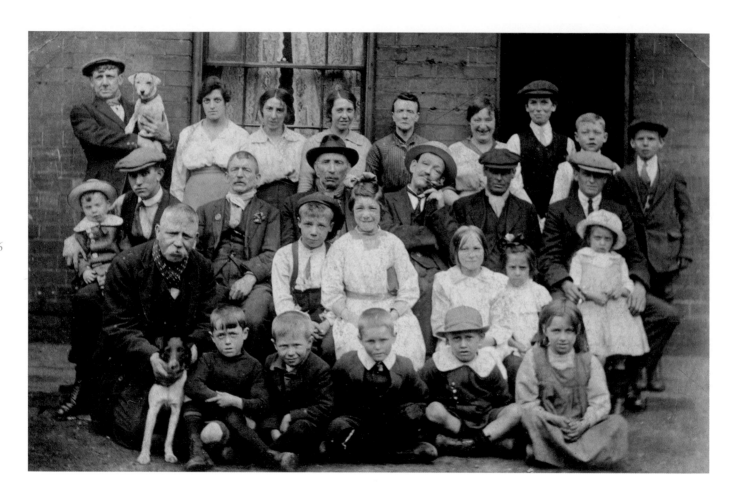

British

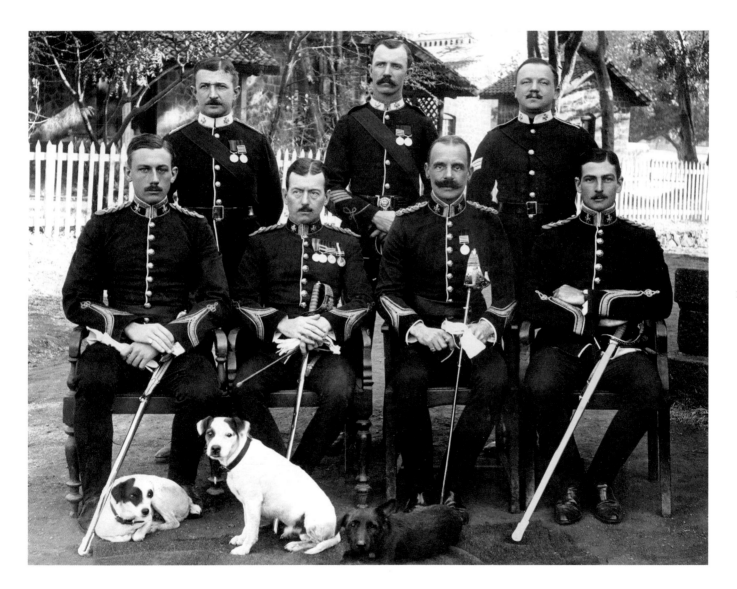

British in India

Album page: Staff Deolali. Back row L to R:
Sgt Chambers, Q.M.S. Thorpe, Q Sgt Milward.
Front row: Lt Dobbie, Brt Major Phelps,
Capt Castle, Lt Chambers.

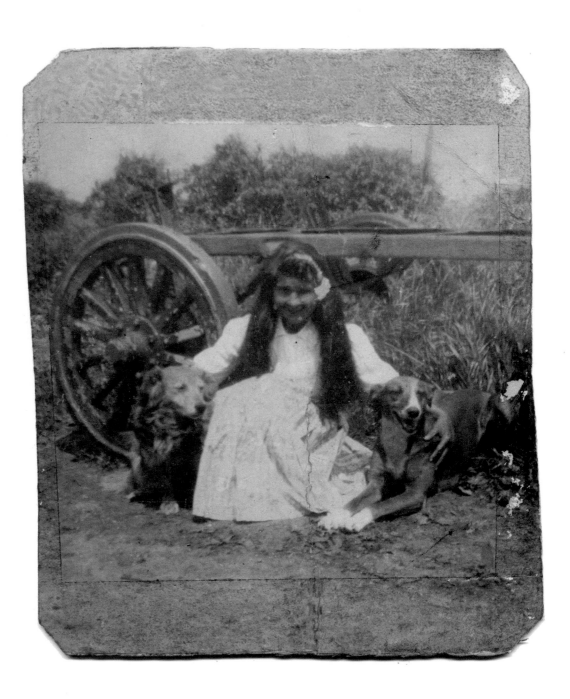

128

British

Note with photograph:
'Mother taken in
Cottrells field'

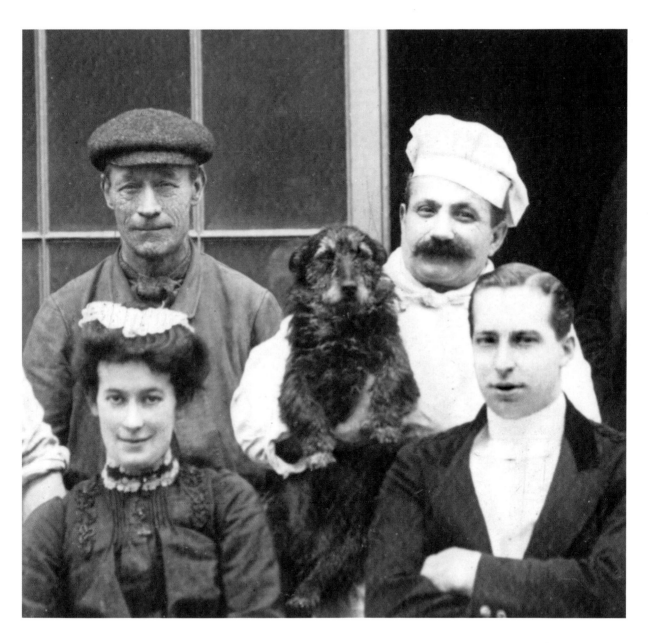

British

Detail from a group of sixteen
household servants.

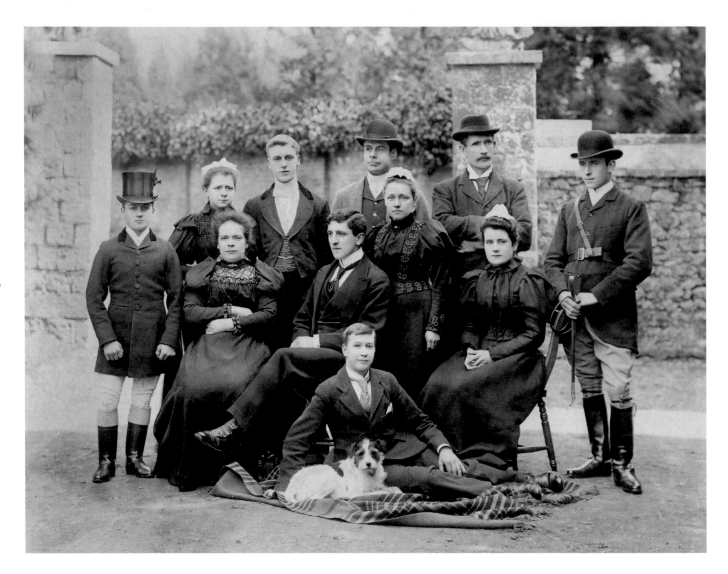

British

(Opposite) British

Miss Isabel Jay: a D'Oyly Carte star in many
of Gilbert and Sullivan's Savoy Operas.

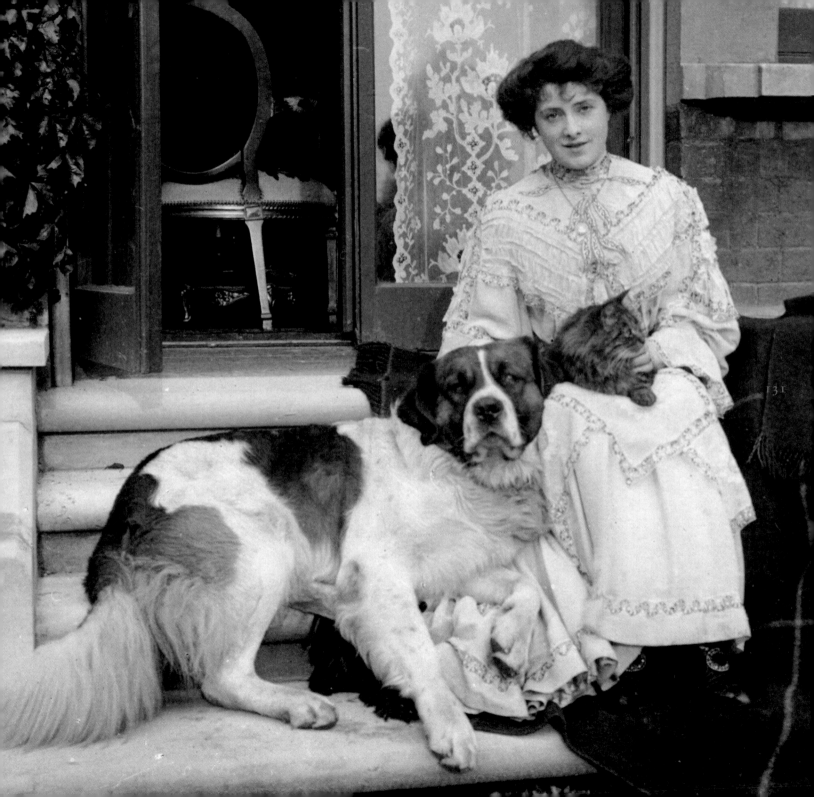

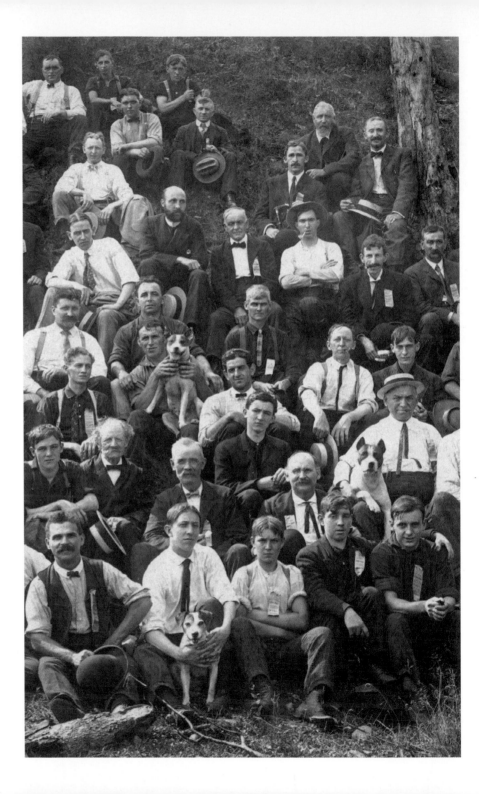

American

Detail from a larger print of seventy men. Note at the bottom: 'Clambake. Wood Department. July 21st 1906.'

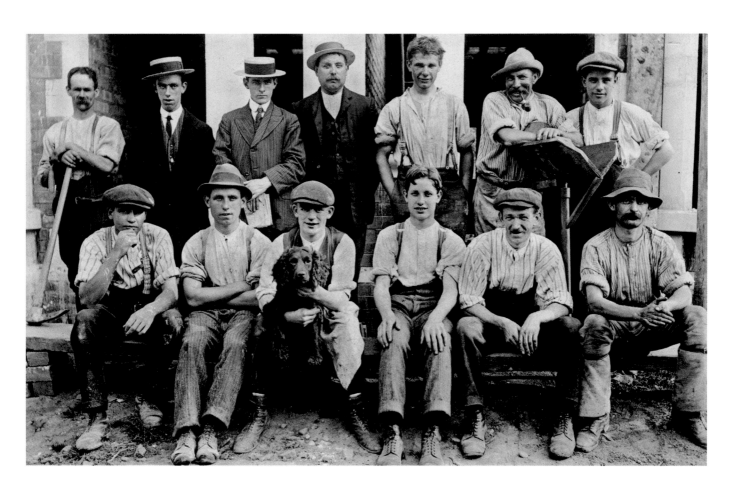

British

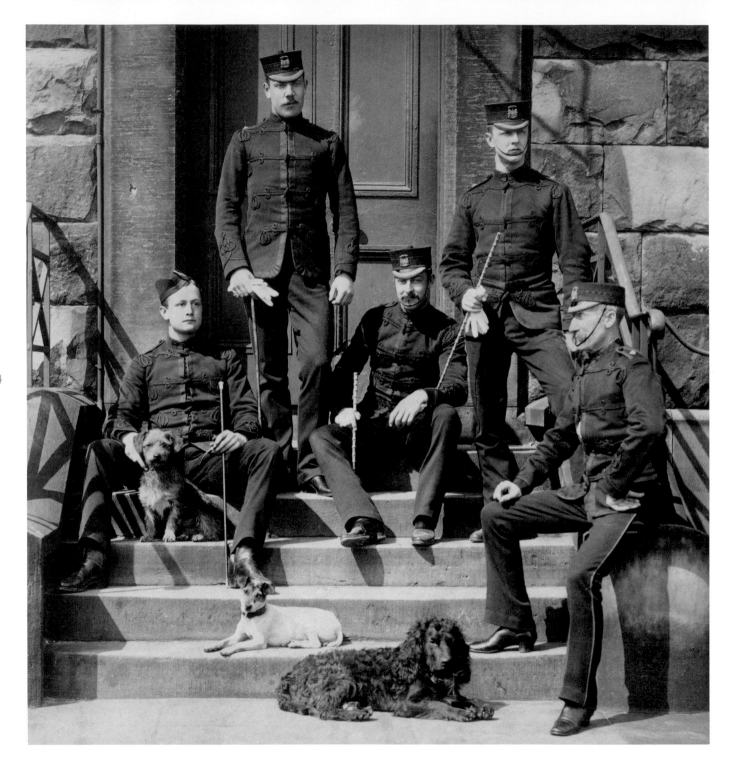

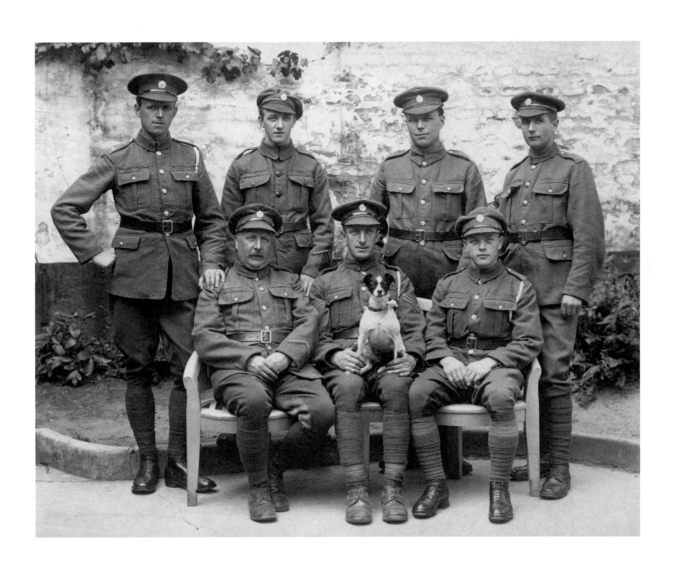

(Opposite) British

Note on reverse: 'Preston
Barracks – 1886.'

British

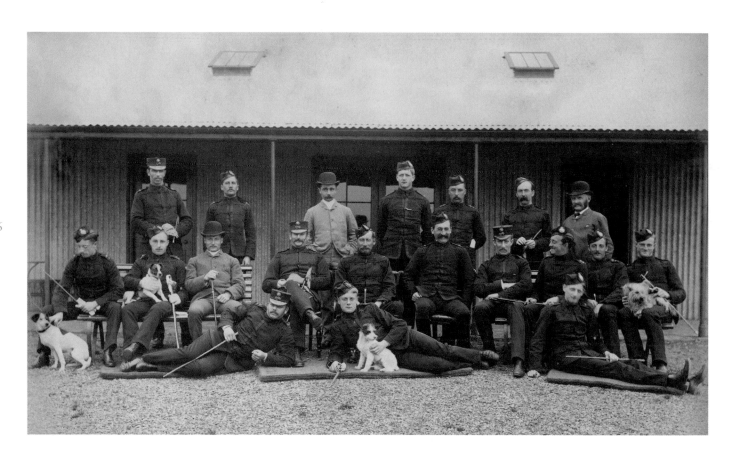

British

Worcestershire regiment.

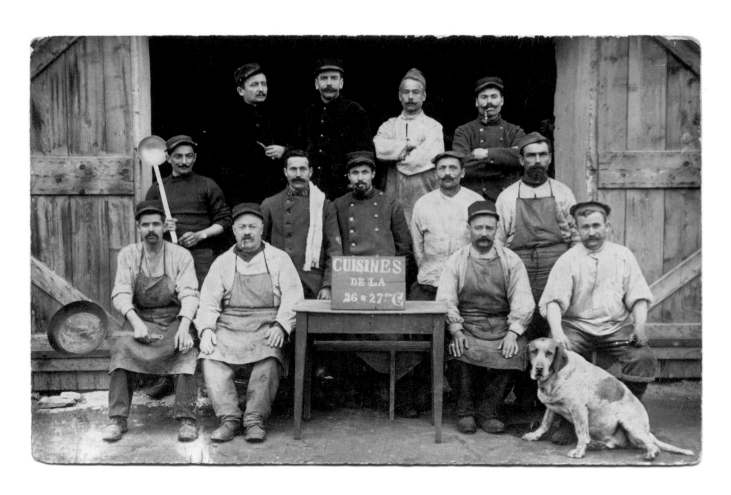

French

Circa 1905 – 1910

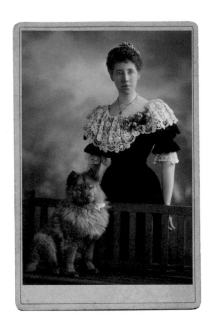

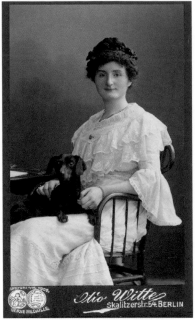

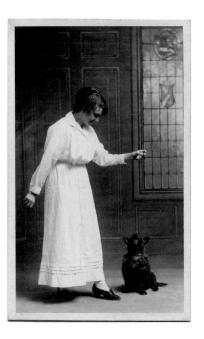

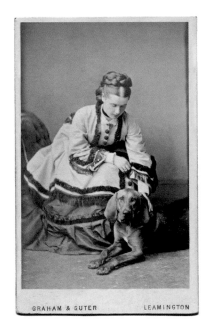

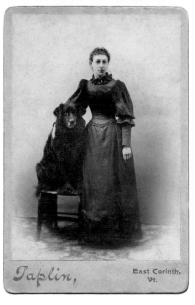

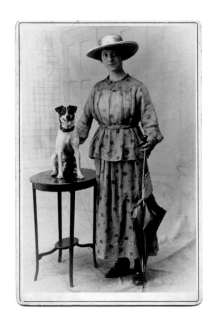

British   German   British

British   American   British

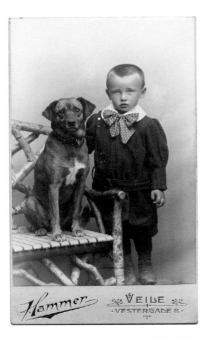

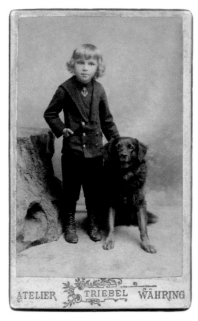

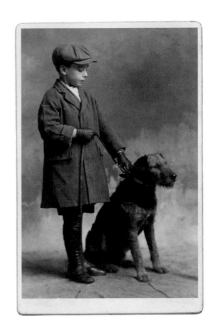

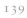

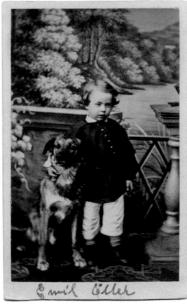

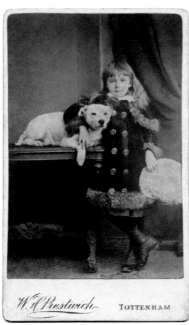

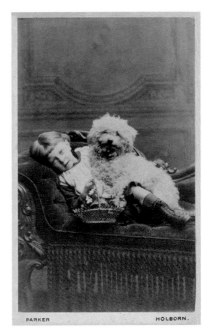

Norwegian

Austrian

British

European

British

British

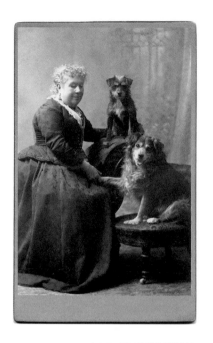

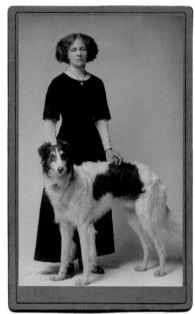

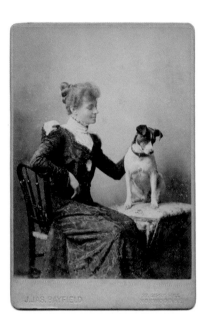

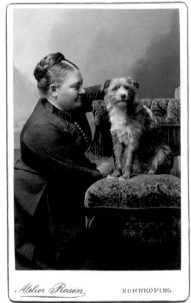

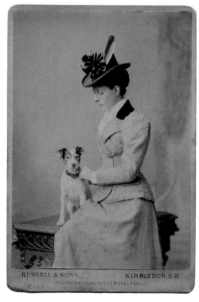

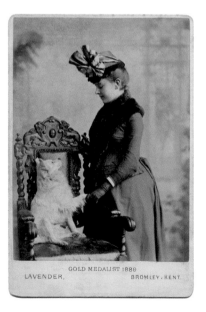

British

Swedish

British

British

British

British

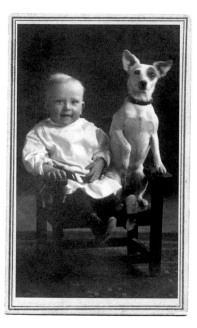

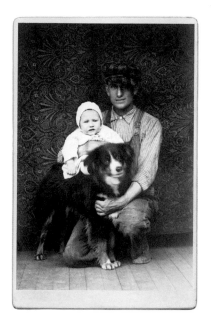

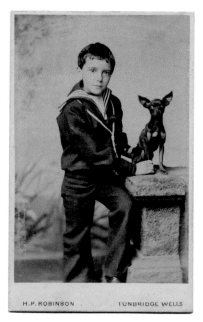

H.P. ROBINSON.   TUNBRIDGE WELLS.

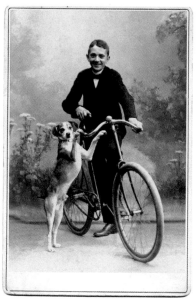

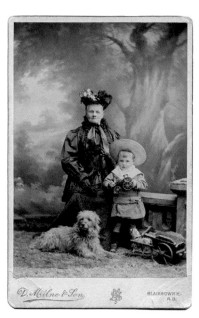

D. Milne & Son   BLAIRGOWRIE, N.B.

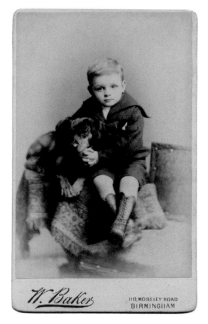

W. Baker   110, MOSELEY ROAD BIRMINGHAM

American
European

American
British

British
British

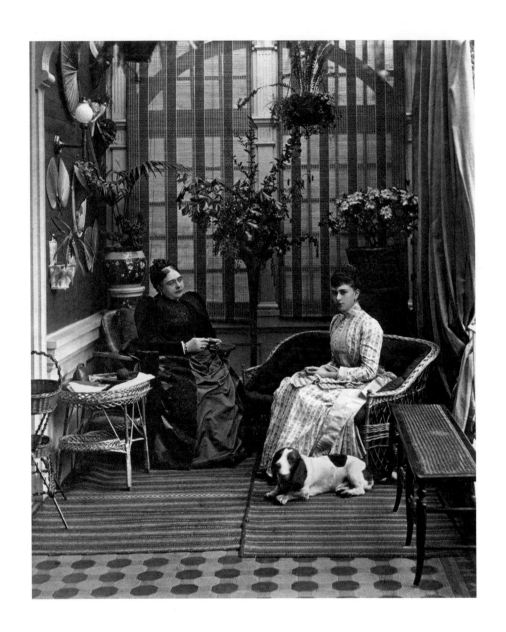

142

British

Princess Mary of Teck (later Queen
Mary) with her mother Princess Mary
Adelaide and Princess Mary Adelaide's
dog Max. 1890.

(opposite)

American

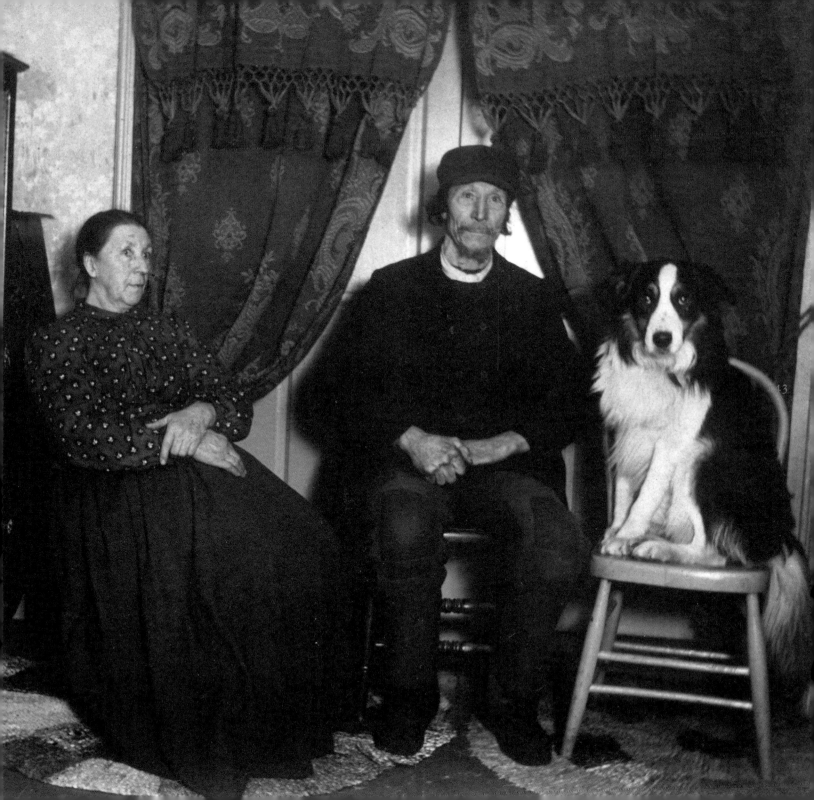

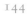

144

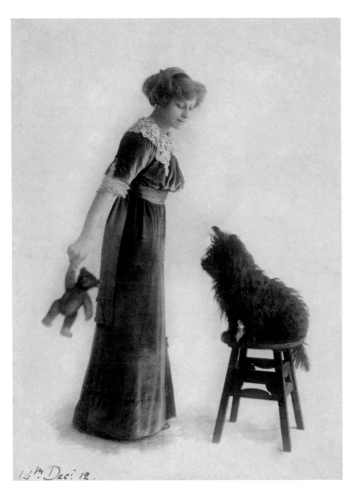

14th Dec: 12.

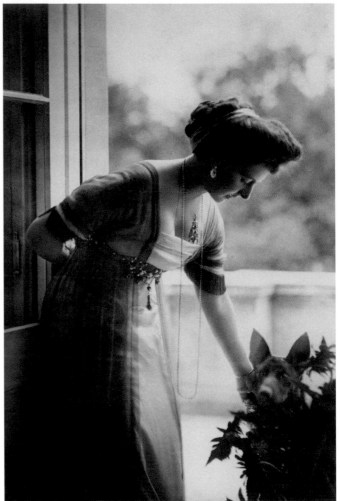

British

Prussian

Princess Eitel Friedrich von Preussen

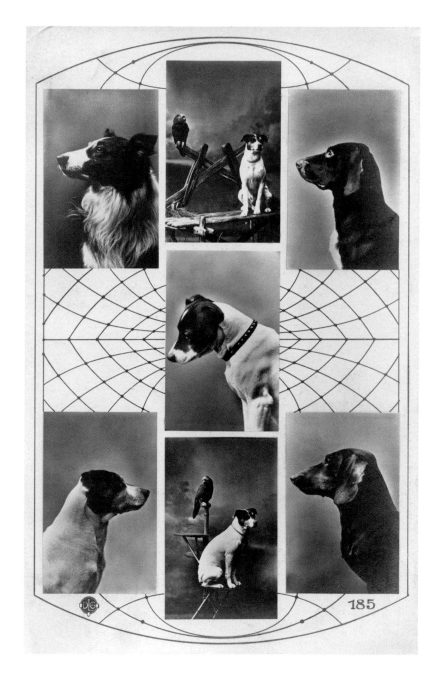

185

Probably European

Perhaps a photographer specialising in images of animals?

146

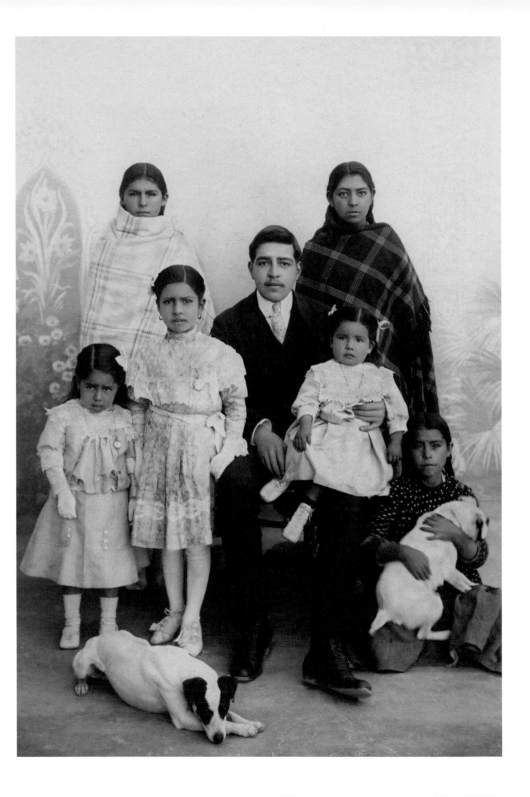

Probably Mexican

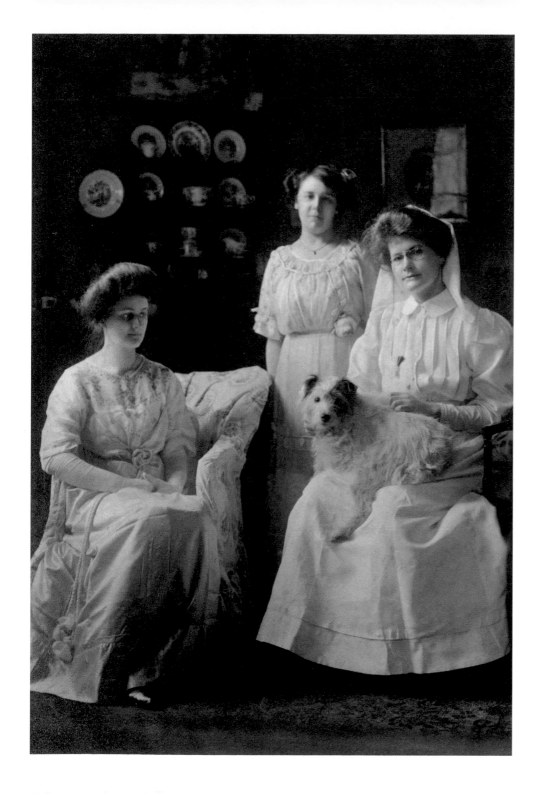

147

British

Note on reverse:
'After the ball. The
self sacrificing one
and the frivolous.'

Further Reading

Early photography

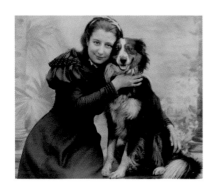

Queen Alexandra.
Queen Alexandra's Christmas Gift Book:
Photographs from my Camera.
London, The Daily Telegraph, 1908.

Cow, Brian and Paul Gates.
The Rise of Popular Photography 1888 – 1939.
London, Ash and Grant, 1977.

Dimond, Frances and Roger Taylor.
Crown and Camera:
The Royal Family and Photography 1842 – 1910.
London, Penguin, 1987.

Frizot, Michel.
A New History of Photography.
Könemann Köln English language edition, 1998.

Harker, Margaret F.
Victorian and Edwardian Photographs.
London, Charles Letts Books, 1975.

Henisch, Heinz and Bridget Henisch.
The Photographic Experience, 1839 – 1914.
The Pennsylvania State University Press, 1994.

Linkman, Audrey.
The Victorians. Photographic Portraits.
London, Tauris Parke Books, 1993.

Sykes, Christopher Simon.
Country House Camera.
London, Pavilion Books, 1980.

Sykes, Christopher Simon.
Country House Album.
The National Trust.
London, Pavilion Books, 1989.

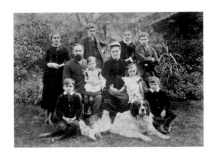

Images of dogs

Carter, Keith.
Bones.
San Francisco, Chronicle Books, 1996.

Eichhorn, Gary and Scott Jones.
The Dog Album.
New York, Stewart, Tabori and
Chang, 2000.

Erwitt, Elliott.
Son of Bitch.
New York, Viking Press, 1974.

Erwitt, Elliott.
Dog Dogs.
London, Phaidon Press, 1998.

Freedman, Jill.
Jill's Dogs.
San Francisco, Pomegranate Artbooks, 1993.

Hall, Libby.
Prince & Others 1850-1940.
London and New York, Bloomsbury, 2000.

Hall, Libby.
Prince & Other Dogs II.
London and New York, Bloomsbury, 2002.

Hall, Libby.
Postcard Dogs.
London and New York, Bloomsbury, 2004.

Mohr, Jean.
Un Chien et son Photographe.
Geneva, Editions Zoé, 1981.

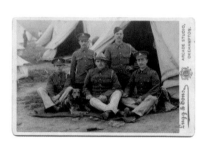

Rosenblum, Robert.
The Dog in Art from Rococo to Post-Modernism.
New York, Harry N. Abrams, 1988.

Scheid, Uwe and Rainer Wick.
Hunde vor der Kamera. Dogs in Focus.
Munich, Weingarten, 1989.

Secord, William.
Dog Painting 1840 – 1940: A Social History of the Dog in Art.
Woodbridge, Suffolk, Antique Collectors' Club, 1992.

Secord, Rosenblum, Rebbert and Bowron.
Best in Show: The Dog in Art from the Renaissance to Today.
New Haven and London, Yale University Press, 2006.

Silverman, Ruth.
The Dog Observed 1844 – 1988.
San Francisco, Chronicle Books, 1988.

Silverman, Ruth.
The Dog.
San Francisco, Chronicle Books, 2000.

Tarry, Ets and Alland.
My Dog Rinty.
New York, Viking Press, 1946.

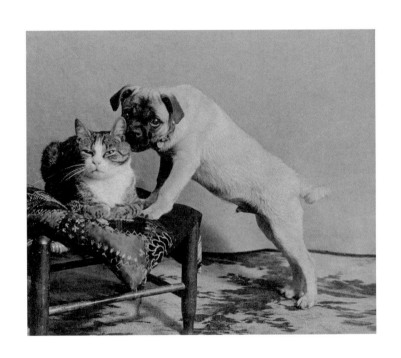

Credits & Formats

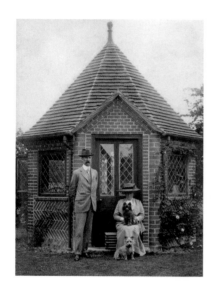

Daguerreotype

p77: photographer not known.

Cartes-de-visite

p101BR, p105L, p105R, p139BL: photographer not known.

p15 Mason and Co. London; p23 G.W. Wilson & Co; p26 W&D Downey; p27L W&D Downey; p27R W&D Downey; p29TC Wm. Hughes. Llangefni; p29TR J. Stodart. Margate; p29BC C. Weidinger; p30TL Hills & Saunders. Cambridge, Oxford, Eton, Harrow & London; p30TC J.P. Starling. High Wycombe; p48TL A Nicholls. Cambridge; p48TC W. Birell. Quarry St, Hamilton; p48TR Franck, Place de la Bourse; p48BR C.S. Cork. Hadleigh Suffolk; p50BR H.H. Reeves. Cleveland Ohio; p51BR RR Boning. St-Leonards-on-sea; p63R Vve Lèon. Roubaix; p66TL Mayall. Brighton; p66TR Alfred Harman. Surbiton Hill; p66BL George Waters. Windermere; p67TL C.V. Bark. Clifton; p67BC Michell & Son. Cornwall; p71 George Bruce. N.B; p74TC G.D. Morse. San Francisco; p74BC W. Clayton. Nottingham; p74BR Lambert Weston & Son. Folkestone; p75TR Thos. Bromwich; p75BC G. Smart. Stirling; p75BR V. Barsokevitsch; p100TL Ch. DeTrez et Simon; p100TC Disderi. 6 Bd des Italiens; p100TR Fred Thurston. Luton; p100BL Universelle. Paris; p101TC A.Weiner. Wien; p101TR Macy. Salisbury; p101BC W. Cooper. Birmingham; p107T G. Th. Hase & Sohn. Freiburgh; P107B Atelier Apollo. Helsinki; p118TC A. Osipoff. Plevna; p118BL F. Hangen. Hassfurt; p119TL T. Vipond. Grantham; p119TC W&D Downey; p119TR Henry J. Cobbold. Hastings; p119BL Gael. Exmouth; p119BC Ainsworth & Dauncey. West of England; p119BR Olsommer. Neuchatel; p138TC Otto Witte. Berlin; p138BL Graham & Suter. Leamington; p139TL Veile. Vestergade 8; p139TC Triebel; p139BC W.H. Prestwich. Tottenham; p139BR W.A. Parker. Holborn; p140BL C. Rosén p141TR H.P. Robinson. Tunbridge Wells; p141BR W. Baker. Birmingham.

Ambrotypes

p76, p78, p79, p80R: photographer not known.

Tintypes

p80L, p81L, p81R: photographer not known.

Stereotypes

p2, p70T, p70B: photographer not known.
p36, p96T Keystone View Company; p131 Rotary.
p151 C.H. Graves. Philadelphia.

Cabinet cards

p135, p148: photographer not known.

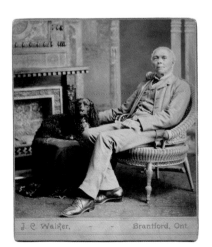

p12 G. Sanders. Bladon. Oxon; p16 Symonds & Co. Portsmouth;
p28TC Elite; p28BL J Browning Exeter; p28BC H. W. Rich. Willimantic
Conn; p29TL Ch. Bergamasco; p30TR J. Crowhurst. Forest Hill;
p30BL Hy. Short. Exeter; p49TL Fred. Palmer. Kingston on Thames;
p49TC Otto J. Frank. New York; p49TR E. Lott. Bridgend;
p49BL J.Pottle. Wimborne; p49BR Walter Baker. Birmingham;
p50TL I.S. Tapley. Lewiston; p50BL E. Dann & Son. Redhill;
p50BC H.D. Hall. Bath ME; p51TL Max Steffeur. Berlin; p51TC Geo.
Dean.Rawalpindi & Murree. Punjab. India; p51BL Pittaway & Jarvis.
Ottawa; p51BC F.Schröck; p60 Window & Grove. London; p66TC
Princes Photo Art Studio. Central Falls R.I.; p66BR William Gill.
Colchester; p67BR Carl Siemsen & Sohn. Hamburg; p74TR Fred.
Robinson. Trumansburgh. N.Y.; p75BL Kent & Fenton. Upper Caterham;
p101TL Ralph Starr. Cambridge; p113 C. Lagriffe; p115 McCullagh.
Stockton California; p116TL Atelier Erna. Frankfurt: p116TR Gustav
Schubert. Wien; p116BL Wilhelm Mann. Salzburg; p116BR W.H. Theaker.
Markdale Ont; p118TL von Ayx. Mainz; p123 H.Hocking& Co.
Birmingham; p138BC Taplin. East Corinth Vt; p140TL Holden, Brighton;
p140TR J. Jas Bayfield. Gipsy Hill, Norwood SE;

p140BC Russell & sons. Wimbledon; p140BR Lavender. Bromley, Kent; p141BC D. Milne and Son. Blairgowrie. p150 Arcade Studio. Oakhampton.

On postcard stock

p13, p14, p18, p21, p22, p28TL, p28TR, p29BL, p31TL, p31TC, p31BL, p31BC, p32, p35, p37, p38, p40, p46, p47, p50TC, p50TR, p52L, p54R, p57L, p57R, p58L, p59L, p62T, p63B, p65TL, p65TR, p65B, p67TR, p68, p69, p75TC, p82, p83, p85, p87, p88, p89, p92, p96B, p97, p99, p100BC, p100BR, p106, p111R, p112, p117L, p117R, p118BC, p122, p126, p133, p137, p138TR, p141TC, 141BL, p143, p145, p152, p156: photographer not known.

p28BR J. Cook. Kilmarnock; p30BC S.S. Wheeler. New York; p30BR the Philco publishing co. London; p31TR W. R. Wilcockson. Holloway Road N; p31BR Elliott's Studios. North Shields; p34 F.H. Biddle. Warwickshire; p41 Kingsway Real Photo; p43 Renard. Baccarat; p44 J.C. Ruddock. Alnwick; p49BC Smithson. Shildon; p52R Ferd. Urbahns. Kiel; p53L H.B. Cooper. Leicester; p55L A. Corbett. Baker St; p55R W&D Downey. Rotary; p56R R. Guilleminot. Paris; p58R Julietta; p59R Lytton & Co. Sheffield; p61 Rotary; p64T Leroy. Draguignon; p64B Leroy. Draguignon; p66BC F. Sharp. Trafalgar Rd Greenwich, by special appointment to the Admiralty; p67TC Eastbourne Photographic. Clapham Common; p72 C.C. Slack & Co. Sioux Falls D.D.; p74TL Cavendish Studios. Eastbourne; p74BL C. Rossillon. Paris; p75TL B. Bing. Anstalt nur Wien; p101BL Maurice Howard. The Portrait Specialist, Leicester, Nottingham, Burslem, Coventry, Liverpool; p102 Julien Freres. Geneve; p103 Julien Freres. Geneve; p104R C.H. Price. Croydon; p108 Myers-Cope Co. 1521 & 1635 Boardwalk, Atlantic City. N.J.; p109 Judges; p111L Rotary Photo; p114 Associated Screen News. Montreal; p118TR C. Mader; p118BR Carl Cloud. Manchester and Bolton; p138BR Jno Emberson. Wimbledon, Surbiton & Tooting; p139TR W. Pearce. High St Lewisham; p140TC Mora Ltd. Elm Grove, Southsea; p141TL Chas Libby; p144R Gust. Liersch & Co. Berlin; p147 Chas. Fearnsides. Penrith.

Prints in other formats

p17, p19, p29BR, p33, p39TL, p39TR, p42, p45L, p45R, p48BC, p53R, p54L, p56L, p63TL, p73, p84, p86, p90, p91, p93, p95, p110T, p110BL, p110BR, p120, p121, p124, p125, p127, p128, p129, p132, p134, p136, p144L, p146: photographer not known.

p20 Queen Alexandra; p25 Hills and Saunders; p39B Peter Eddy. Fabyan House. N.H; p48BL Debenham. Gloucester; p51TR Huebner. Rutherford; p62B The Wykeham Studios Ltd. London; p67BL The deCeru Studio. Huntington Indiana; p94 Goetz; p98 Gulmez Freres. Constantinople; p104L Levi Moore. Albany N.Y; p130 C. Essenhigh Corke. FRPC. Sevenoaks; p138 TL Whitlock. Birmingham and London; p141 Russell & Sons. Baker St. p149 W.H. Woolliscroft. Pontefract; p153 J.C. Walker. Brantford. Ontario.

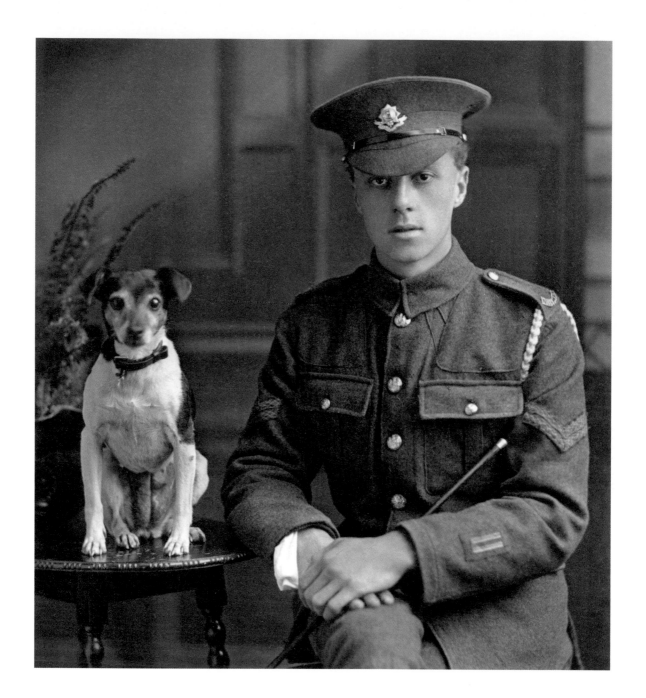

Acknowledgements

First and foremost my thanks to Alexandra Pringle, and to everyone at Bloomsbury who has supported this book from start to finish.

Without the help and advice of my ever-patient husband Tony Hall this book would not have been possible; while many of the American photographs could not have been included without the transatlantic backup of my brother Bill Osborne.

Finally, my thanks to Mike Atkinson, David Cripps, Grenville Collins, Paul Frecker, Brad Feuerhelm, Jesamine Kelly, Jean McKercher, Norman Palmer, Debra Jane Seltzer, Sean Weir and all those many individuals who have so generously shared their knowledge with me, or given me photographs to add to the collection.

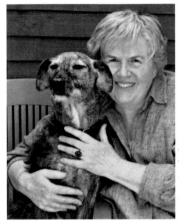

Photograph by Tony Hall

A note on the author

A former press photographer, Libby Hall began collecting dog photographs in the 1960s. Her books *Prince and Other Dogs*, *Prince and Other Dogs II*, *Postcard Dogs* and *Postcard Cats* (with Tom Phillips) are also published by Bloomsbury. She lives in London.

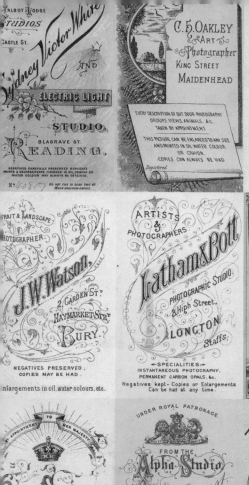
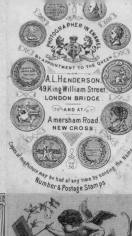
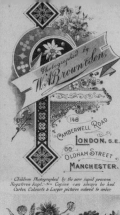
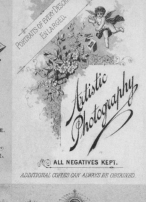
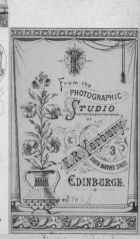
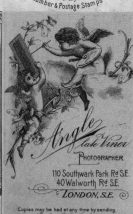
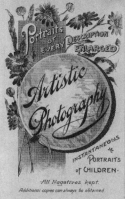
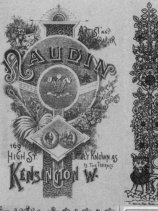
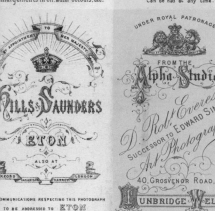
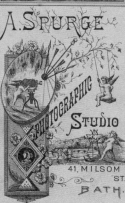
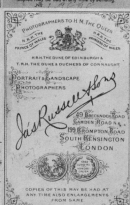
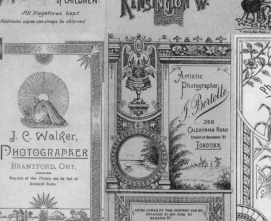
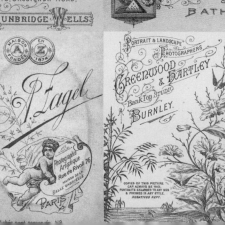
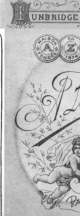
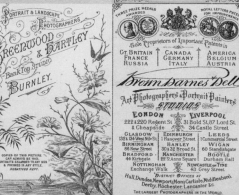
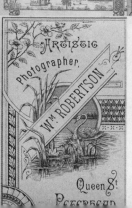
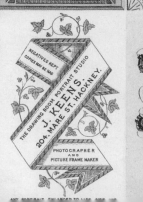